THE
BREAST
BOOK

THE
BREAST
BOOK

DR. MIRIAM STOPPARD

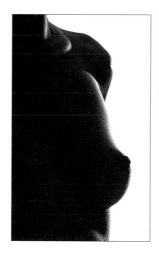

Random House of Canada
Toronto

For Ed, Ed, Hazie, Jude, Eleanor, Sabiha, Doris, and Gwyn

A DK PUBLISHING BOOK

Created and produced by
CARROLL & BROWN LIMITED
5 Lonsdale Road
London NW6 6RA

First Canadian Edition, 1996
1 3 5 7 9 10 8 6 4 2
Published in Canada by
Random House of Canada, Toronto.

Managing Editor Denis Kennedy
Art Director Chrissie Lloyd

Project Editor Theresa Reynolds
Assistant Editors Melanie Halton, Laura Price
US Editors Constance M. Robinson, Kate Zentall

Art Editor Sally Powell
Designer Karen Sawyer

Photography Debi Treloar, Ian Boddy

Production Wendy Rogers

US Consultant Dr. Rache Simmons

First published in Great Britain in 1996
by Dorling Kindersley Limited,
9 Henrietta Street, London WC2E 8PS
Copyright © 1996 Dorling Kindersley Limited
Text copyright © 1996 Miriam Stoppard

Canadian Cataloging-in-Publication Data
Stoppard, Miriam
The breast book

Includes index.
ISBN 0-679-30779-6

1. Breast. 2. Breast – Care and hygiene.
3. Breast – Cancer – Popular works. I. Title.
RG491.S76 1996   618.1'9   C95-932722-3

Reproduced by Colourscan, Singapore
Printed and bound in Great Britain by Butler & Tanner

AUTHOR'S ACKNOWLEDGMENTS

Professional medical help, always important to me in
writing a book, has been unhesitatingly given. Professor Robert
Mansel of University Hospital, Cardiff, and Professor Robert
Rubens of Guy's Hospital, London, have read my text and
nudged it in the direction of a consensus scientific view,
something I could not have done myself. The radiologist Dr.
Eleanor Moskovic of the Royal Marsden Hospital, London,
introduced me to the intricacies of diagnosis by imaging, and
gave me one of the most thrilling moments of the year when I
and her patient watched her put a needle into a breast cyst under
ultrasonic guidance to diagnose and treat a benign condition
in one move before our very eyes. Dr. John Sloane and Mr.
Meirion Thomas of the Royal Marsden Hospital brought me up
to speed on the histopathology and surgery of breast disease. Mr.
James Frame made sure that the plastic surgery section is up to
date. Mr. Ian Fentiman and Dr. David Tong of Guy's Hospital,
along with Professor Rubens, were good enough to show me
how a really great breast unit works and charitably clear my
befuddled mind. I and all my readers are the beneficiaries of
their wisdom and generosity.

Friends have opened up vistas for me, particularly Dr. Judith
Collins on the breast in art, and Sir Eduardo Paolozzi on the
breast as a modern icon.

This is the first book I've written with help from my family:
my youngest son, Ed, gamely took up a vacation job from his
university to act for a while as my researcher and gained
notoriety among his friends as an expert on all things mammary.
With my sister Hazel, an ex-editor, I had that rare feeling of
being in safe hands. Not only were her analyses of sociological
questions searching and illuminating, they were larded with
delicious turns of phrase and dry wit that I could not resist.
I'm indebted to Ed and Hazel.

Miriam Stoppard

FOREWORD

Dr. Miriam Stoppard is well known for her contribution to public education on matters of health care, both as an author and as a media presenter. *The Breast Book* not only focuses on health issues but goes further with accounts of many facets of the history and sociology of the breast.

The clear, informative discussion of breast self-examination and screening addresses the needs of women who are eager to take responsibility for their breast health. Individuals who become anxious about what may well be normal changes in their breasts will be greatly reassured by Dr. Stoppard's chapter on benign breast disease.

Nevertheless, the possibility of cancer is a legitimate cause for concern, and women need enough information, written in the kind of accessible everyday language found in this book, to determine when to seek medical attention.

Dr. Stoppard provides a description of breast disease and what is known about its causes. The options of treatment are explained to help a woman evaluate her choices. The importance of appropriate surgery, radiation therapy, and drug treatment for cancer is emphasized.

This unique book will be welcomed by all women, for whom it will provide the essential information to understand breast health and breast disease.

Rache M. Simmons, M.D.
ASSISTANT ATTENDING, BREAST SURGERY
THE NEW YORK HOSPITAL-CORNELL MEDICAL CENTER
DIRECTOR OF THE NEW YORK HOSPITAL-CORNELL BREAST CENTER
ASSISTANT DIRECTOR OF STRANG-CORNELL BREAST CENTER
NEW YORK, NY

CONTENTS

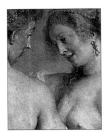
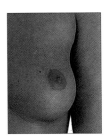
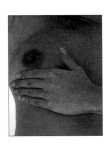
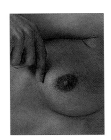
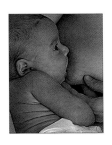

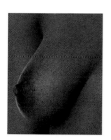

6 Cosmetic Breast Surgery

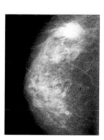

7 Benign Breast Changes

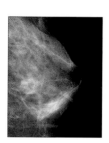

8 Breast Cancer

9 Treating Breast Cancer

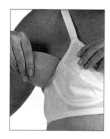

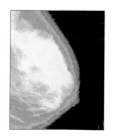

INTRODUCTION

This book is for everyone who has breasts and everyone who loves breasts. For the majority of women, breasts are bound up with self-image, womanhood, and sexuality, but social conditioning being what it is, few women are happy with their breasts. Most men, on the other hand, think their partners' breasts are perfectly lovely, as research shows. This book is not, however, about mastoconcupiscence, though no woman escapes entirely from our society's obsession with breasts. Rather, it is a celebration of breasts through all their vicissitudes.

WHY A BOOK ABOUT THE BREAST?

Pride is something I'd like every woman to feel about her breasts and I hope that after reading this book every woman will. It may be in reading the book that you discover the truly feminine and often erotic pleasure of breastfeeding. And given the importance of breasts to self-image, it may encourage you to take the plunge and investigate cosmetic surgery as part of your right to decide how you look. At the very least I hope the reader will discover some surprising and gratifying facts: that every breast, however small, is capable of successful lactation; that breasts evolved through millions of years of Darwinian adjustment by sexual selection; that the nipple during sexual arousal achieves just as profound an erection as the penis and can cause orgasm.

This book could be seen as a self-help manual because every woman is responsible for the health of her breasts, whether it's finding the right bra to give comfort and support for them or undertaking regular breast self-examination (BSE) to detect any problems.

GETTING TO KNOW YOUR BREASTS

My overriding aim is to make you unafraid of your breasts. Only women can know the anxiety that springs from pain in our breasts – a symptom, incidentally, that almost always rules out anything sinister. In the last few years, however, doctors have come to accept mastalgia as a debilitating condition for which we now have a variety of treatments.

Breasts are far from quiescent: throughout our fertile lives, their glandular tissues ebb and flow with the cyclical surges of our ovarian hormones, sometimes swelling one whole cup-size in the second half of the month only to die back when menstruation intervenes. Month by month every woman experiences this evidence that her breasts are an integral part of her unique endocrine orchestra.

Breasts can become lumpy with every cycle, and it's normal. You can feel the changes in your breasts through your menstrual cycle by doing regular BSE. Most newly discovered lumps are harmless. Scientists have made great strides in understanding benign breast lumps, and lumps that in the past were surgically removed are now recognized as nothing more than the natural expression of the breast's development.

The female breast goes on maturing until menopause, and its different elements mature in turn. In our early 20s, the lobules are growing, and a lobule can turn quite normally into a lump called a fibroadenoma, sometimes as large as a lemon but nonetheless harmless. In our 30s and 40s it's the turn of the glands, and so we get cysts, firm to the touch but hardly ever malignant. Toward the end of our fertile lives the milk ducts begin to age and so we are prone to nipple problems. Once we are aware of these normal phases of growth and shrinkage, we are liberated from fear and empowered to act.

PUTTING BREAST CANCER IN PERSPECTIVE

Breast cancer takes up a major portion of this book. I have aimed to demystify it because I believe that in understanding it we can manage it. We shouldn't allow the fear of breast cancer to tyrannize our lives.

For every lump in the breast that turns out to be cancerous, 10 others are benign and harmless. For every 10 women with a cancerous lump, 6 or 7 will be treated without removal of the breast, and for 3 or 4 the cause of death will be something other than cancer. If you are prepared to take the initiative so that your lump is diagnosed and treated early, you will be one of the 85 percent of women who will be alive and well for a minimum of five years after diagnosis.

The longer you live, the less chance you have of dying of breast cancer. By the time you're in your middle 60s your chances of dying from a heart attack are four times greater, while your chances of dying from breast cancer are about half of what they were at 50. So although the chances of getting breast cancer may increase as we age, the chances of dying from it diminish with every successive year.

REDUCING YOUR RISK

Informing ourselves of the causes of breast cancer can greatly improve our chances of avoiding and defeating it. Knowledge of risk factors can help you to reduce your own risk with life choices, such as having your first baby before 30 rather than after if you can, and lifestyle changes such as keeping your weight down, which seems to be more important than the actual diet you eat.

A family history of breast cancer is far and away the risk that should concern you most. Women with such a background should seek counseling in their 20s. The more affected relatives you have and the younger they were when they developed cancer, the greater the risk. Women belonging to breast-cancer families, where a potent gene is probably at work, are at greatest risk and should be monitored frequently so that expeditious action can be taken if necessary.

Whatever our personal risk, there are two methods of screening open to all of us – BSE and mammography – and we should take advantage of both. I could not be anything but an advocate of BSE, whether it's proved to detect cancer earlier or not, because it promotes breast awareness. It makes us feel at home with our own bodies, so it's easier

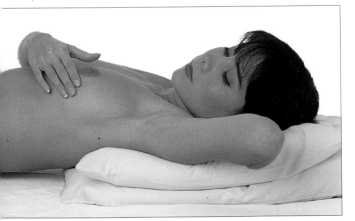

to consult a doctor about anything untoward, rather than just hoping it will go away. Mammography has its advocates and its detractors, but it would be a brave oncologist who abandoned a screening program given that screening has meant that smaller, easier-to-treat tumors now outnumber large, difficult-to-treat tumors. Having examined the worldwide evidence on the usefulness of mammography, I come down firmly on the side of screening.

KEEPING A GRIP

No woman remains untouched by finding a new lump in her breast or having a suspicious shadow show up on a mammogram. Your complex psychological reactions will affect not only your health but also your relationships, lifestyle, and body image. You don't have to shoulder this burden alone. There are many sources of help available, particularly the nurse counselors on the staff of every breast center. Knowing this, I implore every woman to

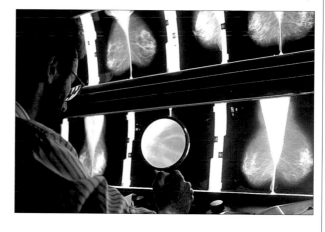

report breast symptoms early. Don't procrastinate. While it would be unnatural not to be anxious, it would be irrational to panic. The chances are overwhelmingly that whatever you've found is not cancer. But, most important, if it *is* cancer and you seek a diagnosis quickly so that it's caught early, the probability of a cure is high. As more and more women are getting treatment earlier, it's now quite common to meet a woman admitting she had cancer 15 or more years ago.

THE GOOD NEWS

I want every woman to know about special breast centers where you will get a rapid and precise diagnosis using techniques at the forefront of medical technology. Some even provide a one-stop, 24-hour diagnosis. A whole team of doctors including an oncologist, a surgeon, a radiotherapist, a pathologist, a radiologist, and a nurse counselor will consider your individual case, and you'll get personalized treatment. A most important aspect of this team effort is that you and your family will be included in the discussion, and all the options for treatment will be put to you and carefully explained. Your preferences will be given emphasis and your rights as a breast cancer patient respected. It's your right to seek referral to and a second opinion from a breast center.

Be assured that you do have time for a second opinion. The age when surgeons acted in haste to remove a breast has passed. Of course breast cancer must be treated promptly, but promptly with the best solution. We no longer see breast cancer as an emergency. There is time to see another doctor, have special tests, ask questions, and consult your family and loved ones. This is why you no longer have to give permission for a mastectomy when you go in for a biopsy; it is safe for you and your doctor to take the time to decide on treatment after the results of the biopsy are known. All this gives you the best chance of a cure.

THE LATEST TREATMENTS

It is no longer necessary to equate breast cancer with losing a breast. In the past ten years, surgery for breast cancer has changed dramatically. The aim now is to conserve the breast whenever possible and mastectomy has been safely replaced with lumpectomy for many women. The choice will be yours, because, with modern methods for assessing breast cancer and statistically proven treatment regimens aimed at killing both the tumor and any "seedlings" that may have escaped, there are always several equally effective possibilities.

Nowadays nearly all women with breast cancer will receive some sort of adjuvant systemic therapy – that is, hormones or chemotherapy – which aims to kill any cancer cells that have escaped from the primary tumor and settled elsewhere in the body. Researchers have been testing different chemotherapy treatments for years to reach our present state of sophistication. And with the advent of tamoxifen we have discovered an agent that reduces mortality by a third and also protects postmenopausal women from heart attacks and osteoporosis and may even prevent breast cancer in high-risk women.

Your doctors are just as concerned about the quality of life after treatment as you are. Those women who do need a mastectomy are no longer condemned to living with unsightly scars. Reconstruction of your breast can be done as part of the mastectomy or months later. Implants are available, or your own tissue may be used to refashion a breast similar in every way to your other.

In the light of all this I sincerely hope that any reader contracting breast cancer will feel there's reason for hope. At no time has there been such precision of diagnosis, care, and treatment. Never before have we had the tools at our disposal to give every woman individualized treatment down to cellular level. And the first step rests with you. Women are fortunate in a way that men aren't. We can feel our breasts and detect changes; no man can check his own prostate gland. The second step requires courage, fortitude, and stoicism – but then women have always possessed these qualities.

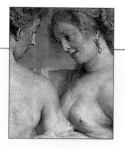

CHAPTER ONE

MYTHS AND REALITIES

From the earliest civilizations, the
breast has been a tremendously potent
image of womankind. Through war
and peace, fashion, religion, art, and
literature, it has been revered, praised,
lusted after, reviled, and exploited.
A powerful representation of beauty,
the breast remains a most compelling
symbol of our femininity.

HISTORY AND FASHION

Over the last 6,000 years – ever since human beings started to write their own stories and leave purposeful records of themselves – the human shape has remained essentially the same. At any given time, however, a particular build and shape has been prized above others – that is to say, it has been fashionable. Quite why our species is driven by a desire to change the way we look on a fairly regular basis is unclear. There is no denying that though we may not know what it is that drives us, driven we are to beautify and re-create ourselves in the image of whatever the current fashion dictates. For women all over the world, the breast has always been a prominent fashion item.

THE IDEAL TYPE

Works of art and other pictorial records can tell us a great deal about changing fashions in breasts and their display. If we look at the way people have been depicted in art forms over the centuries, however, we often have to bear in mind that what is shown, particularly if it is not a personal portrait, may be an idealized type rather than the norm. Rubens painted large, fleshy, dimpled women not because most seventeenth-century Flemish women were like that, but because that shape was fashionable at the time. The flapper girls of the 1920s were not uniformly flat-chested; these women wore undergarments that constricted and flattened their busts because that was regarded as the ideal shape during that particular period.

THE VENUS FIGURINES

The earliest depictions of women date from some 25,000 years ago. They are carved in stone, mammoth ivory, and clay, and measure 1½–8½ inches (4–22 centimeters) in height; the majority are at the lower end of the range. More than 60 of these figurines have been found over a large area of Europe. Virtually all the figurines have huge breasts, thighs, abdomens, and hips, but

Changing ideals
When Rubens painted
The Three Graces *in the seventeenth century, he gave them rounded, fleshy figures, reflecting the favored body shape of that time.*

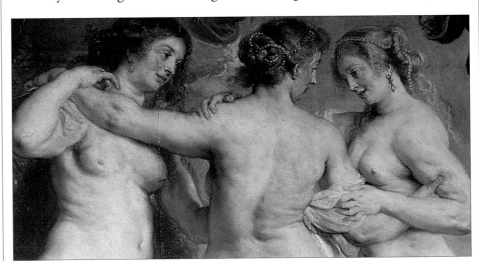

their other features are sketchy. They have been interpreted in various ways: a common view is that they are fertility symbols, which is why they are often called Venus figurines, since Venus is the Roman goddess of love. Whether they were objects of worship or talismans for women who wished to become pregnant, though, is not known.

We can be certain that they are not simply figurines of obese women. It is unlikely that obesity was common in the hunter-gatherer societies that produced these figures; obesity requires a settled life, domestication of plants and animals, and not too much in the way of labor.

It therefore seems likely that such figurines signified the breeding and suckling functions of women. Pregnancy and lactation usually bring enlargement of those parts of the body that seem so very exaggerated in the figurines. Large breasts and bellies are characteristic of pregnant women, and fat develops on their upper arms and thighs to provide for the extra energy costs of lactation (see p.82). The female reproductive function has almost always been venerated, even in the more male-dominated societies, so these exaggerated representations of fertile women represented an ideal in their culture.

BARE-BREASTED WOMEN

Even in cultures where today it is usual to hide the breast, the naked breast has appeared fairly regularly throughout history. It is not always possible to decide whether this is because it was a feature of formal or ceremonial dress, or whether the breast was specifically displayed in order to attract the attention of others within the society.

Ancient civilizations Among the most celebrated images of women from early civilizations are those of the Minoan snake goddesses of Crete, dating from between 2000 and 1500 B.C. They are generally shown with snakes entwined around their arms, waists, and headdresses; their bodices are specifically fashioned to display their bare breasts. This mode of dress may, however, have been confined to women with religious roles rather than worn by the majority simply for reasons of fashion.

In ancient Egypt, the breasts were commonly displayed even though they were not, strictly speaking, bared completely. Many pictures of women dressed for formal occasions, such as banquets, show that they often wore garments of extremely fine linen, which was just as transparent as today's flimsier fabrics. Every feature of the upper body was clearly meant to be visible.

Europe In seventeenth- and eighteenth-century Europe, the bared or grossly accentuated breast occasionally became fashionable. In the 1770s, dresses were fitted with structures of wire and cork to exaggerate the rounded fleshiness of the breasts and bottom. This fashion was quickly followed, as is often the case, by its antithesis. In Napoleon's time, women wore loose dresses made of diaphanous fabrics

Mother goddess
The earliest representations of the human form date from as long as 25,000 years ago and show women with exaggerated breasts. These are believed to have been symbols of fertility.

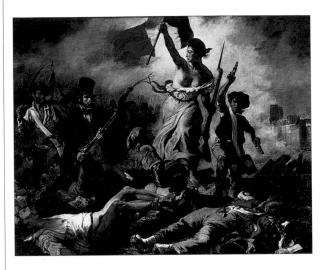

On the battlefield
The figure of Liberty in Delacroix's painting Liberty Leading the People *is a famous example of the bare-breasted woman shown as a powerful rather than an erotic figure.*

through which the breasts were clearly visible – characterizing the Empire look. Such styles were confined to the rich women of the aristocracy; they were not compatible with the manual labors of the poorer working women.

Visible breasts were considered to be extremely offensive by some, including this anonymous man writing in 1694: "This laying out of naked breasts is a temptation to Sinne. Those who have their garments made on such a fashion, that their necks and breasts are in great part left naked . . . invite customers, by setting open their Shop windows."

In Victorian times, female semi-nudity was quite acceptable in art. So long as a drapery or two covered the pudenda, the breasts were quite often left bare. The drapery suggested classical art, and that was equated with a high moral tone. The fashionable Victorian woman herself, despite our notions of that era as being one of sexual repression, would have displayed acres of bosom in her formal evening wear.

THE POWERFUL BREAST

The bare-breasted woman as a symbol of power, particularly of the power to inspire, has frequently been used by artists – quite often in situations where bare-breasted women were least likely to be found, such as the battlefield (Boudicca being a dramatic exception).

Bared breasts and battlefields have a long and close association. Delacroix's *Liberty Leading the People* provides a good example. Liberty is represented as a stirring woman, exhorting the men around her to carry on the fight.

On the field, breasts are best placed to inspire, as they are something of a hindrance in battle. The Greeks told tales of the Amazons, female warriors who were said to cut off one of their breasts so that they could wield their bows more effectively. Another famous female warrior, Joan of Arc, went only so far as to cover her female shape with men's clothing.

One of the most powerful of all bare-breasted women is Marianne, the symbol of France. Unlike Britannia, she does not sit sedately, holding spear and shield and obviously hoping to have her portrait painted; rather she strides through or hovers over battlegrounds *"pour encourager les autres."* For the French revolutionaries, Marianne came to epitomize the total woman: not only did she rally and lead the troops, she fed them. Her bared breasts were seen as lactating; her breast milk fed the masses. Indeed, there are statues of Marianne rigged up with tubes that pump milk through the nipples. On a less elevated plane, soldiers in recent times have revered their pinups.

In the last analysis, the breast is a powerful symbol of what is being fought for. To be killed in war is one danger; to have the womenfolk appropriated by the enemy is another. The breast does not fight, but it inspires those who do.

THE BREAST IN RELIGIOUS ART

Throughout history, attitudes toward women, sexuality, and the body have been determined by religious teachings. Although in this century religious doctrine has been rapidly losing its hold on the collective imagination in many parts of the world, old habits die hard. We can therefore find clues to different attitudes to the breast in the art and literature of the world's major religions.

CHRISTIANITY

The two women whose images dominate Western religious art are Eve and the Virgin Mary. They illustrate the ambivalence in Christian attitudes toward women: Eve the fallen woman and Mary the chaste mother. Eve is almost always shown before, or at the moment of, the Fall, and she is almost always therefore naked. Mary is generally shown swathed in drapery and, though feminine, is basically sexless in any earthy sense.

Although she is venerated as the supreme mother, Mary is seldom shown suckling Jesus, and her breasts are hidden as Eve's are visible. An exception to this rule are Tuscan paintings of the fourteenth century onward, many of which portrayed Mary with a bared breast. This is often lacking in realism, however, a problem that has less to do with the artist's ability to represent a breast than with his reticence at portraying the Virgin in any way that might arouse the wrong responses in the viewer. An exception is Ambrogio Lorenzetti's painting *Madonna del Latte* ("The Madonna of Milk"), which is a heartwarmingly realistic depiction with the infant Jesus suckling and holding his mother's breast. An early fifteenth-century painting by an anonymous Florentine painter, *The Intercession of Christ and the Virgin*, shows Mary holding a rather disembodied breast and interceding with the risen Christ on behalf of sinners with the words "Dearest son, because of the milk I gave you, have mercy on them."

The image of the Madonna suckling Jesus is a very affecting one, and it is somewhat surprising that it does not figure a great deal more frequently in Christian religious art. Perhaps it was thought that Eve had already appropriated the breast for more questionable purposes than suckling a baby.

The breast as temptation Women in Western, and predominantly Christian, culture might just have recovered from the second-class status conferred on them by being a by-product of Adam's rib, but

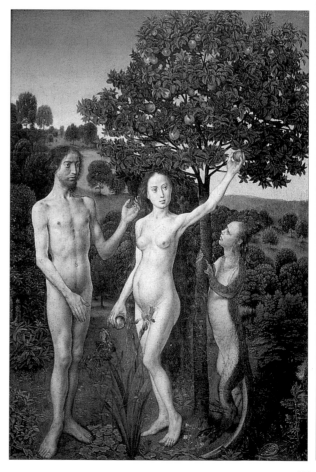

The fallen woman
In this painting of the temptation in the Garden of Eden, the artist makes the shape of Eve's breasts echo the shape of the forbidden fruit, drawing a clear parallel between sexuality and sin.

for the second blow: Eve's role in the fall from grace. Adam is rarely reviled for giving in to temptation, but Eve is everywhere condemned for offering it. The similarity between the apple, which was the lure, and the breast, which was the visible badge of sinful woman, was not lost on artists. In Hans Baldung's *Adam and Eve* (1536), Eve holds the apple and Adam holds Eve's breast. In Masaccio's *Expulsion* (1427), Adam covers his eyes and Eve covers her breasts. When St. Barbara and St. Agnes were martyred, their breasts were first cut off.

The breasts are seen repeatedly, in both the art and literature of the West, as the outward sign of woman's sinfulness, and her sinfulness is most often characterized as lust. What men had first experienced as everything that was good, satisfying, warm, secure, and loving – the mother's breast – they were later taught to scorn as the outward sign of a deadly sin. It is not surprising that women have suffered the consequences of such willful confusion.

It would be naive, however, to see the story of the creation of woman and the fall from grace as the origin of women's woes and men's domination. As with creation myths the world over, its function was to rationalize and justify the social system it professed to inspire. Women were not deemed to be inferior to men because the Bible said that Adam was given dominion over Eve; they were already deemed to be inferior to men, and the Bible merely confirmed this in a particularly powerful way. The price of this convenient myth was the eclipse of any healthy respect for the human body, breasts and all, leaving the female form as a degenerate model of the ideal male body. It is all the more fascinating, therefore, that in recent years science has begun to suggest that, biologically, the female body is the norm, and the male body the variant.

ISLAM

In Arab Islamic culture, the breast does not traditionally have the same importance in calculating female beauty as it does in the West. The thighs, calves, and buttocks are equally valued, and the ideal is that all should be ample. Boyishness in women is not desirable. With the spread of Western books, films, television, and advertising, however, fashions in female beauty are changing, particularly in the large cities.

Islam, even more so than Christianity, has very mixed feelings about the female and her body. Sexual pleasure is regarded as a gift from Allah and is therefore to be enjoyed, but the sexuality and seductiveness of women is also seen as dangerous and to be rigidly controlled. This is why in some Islamic countries women have to cover themselves completely except in the most intimate family settings. The power of female sexuality to seduce men will, if not confined and controlled, lead to disorder and anarchy. Extreme modesty is therefore demanded of a woman, though she too has the right to enjoy sexual fulfillment with her husband. Traditionally, except where her labor was needed in the outside world, as in agricultural work, modesty was enforced by confining a woman to her home. A modern author describes how her grandmother passed through the streets only twice, once to the house of her husband after marriage and the second time to be buried. Nowadays, however, television, video, and billboards display the same voluptuous and carnal images that swamp the Western world, and advertisements for uplifting bras and women in provocative poses are paraded in front of women who themselves may not even lift their eyes to those of a man.

HINDUISM

Hindu culture celebrates the physical; the body is cherished and each part of it is seen as having a role to play in sexual relations. Making love is seen as a way of re-enacting the passion of the Great God Shiva and his wife Parvati.

The Kama Sutra Written some 2,000 years ago, the *Kama Sutra* is one of the cornerstones of the Hindu religion, intended to instruct believers as to how lovemaking can best be done with seriousness and pleasure. It is extremely detailed and was meant to be acted on in its entirety.

The writers of the *Kama Sutra* had a highly accomplished understanding of the sensitivities of the body and recognized that the breast, particularly the nipple, is important in sexual arousal. Three primary methods of stimulating the breast are given: pressing or fondling, scratching, and biting. Depending on which of these is employed, and with what forcefulness or ardor, differing meanings are implied. The marks made by the nails and the teeth are a reminder of pleasure and a token of the passion experienced when husband and wife are reunited. "The love of a woman when she sees the marks of nails on the private parts of her body… becomes again fresh and new." Interestingly, the breasts are referred to as one of the "private parts" of a woman's body, with all that that implies about their responsiveness and sexuality.

Hindu erotic sculpture One of the most refreshing things about Hindu erotic sculpture is that because it is so closely associated with, or rather a part of, religious life, it is public. Anyone approaching the eleventh-century Kandariya Mahadeo temple at Khajuraho in northern India can see immediately that the celebration of divine and human sexuality is central to its builders' belief system. The huge towers are encrusted with stone carvings of immortals and mortals, many of whom are engaged in the most staggering variety of sexual activities – staggering particularly to Westerners, unused to such a display of explicitly sexual acts in a place of worship, perhaps.

These carvings give a clear picture of the type of woman's body that was prized in the culture. The breasts are very large globes and appear high on the chest above a tiny waist and full hips and upper thighs – the direct opposite of the slim, boyish figures with pert breasts that are presently the ideal in Western societies.

Erotic figures
These Hindu temple carvings celebrate the breast in a way that is alien to the Christian and Muslim traditions. Their idealized breast is circular rather than conical and positioned high on the chest.

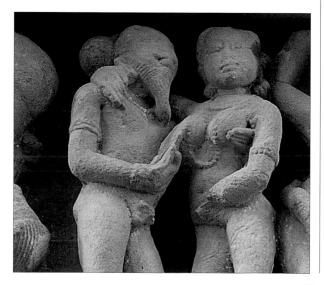

HISTORY OF UNDERWEAR

Only during this century has the idea that breasts need support been widely accepted. Before the existence of the bra, breasts were flattened or emphasized by a variety of undergarments according to the fashion of the day.

De-emphasis In the thirteenth century, women wore short bodices that severely flattened their breasts and full skirts that hung from a raised waistline so as to emphasize the stomach. The fashion for very long and full sleeves also helped to emphasize a slender torso and draw the eye down, away from the breast.

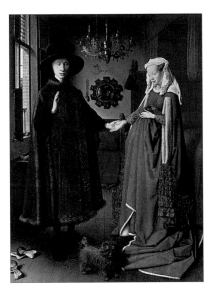

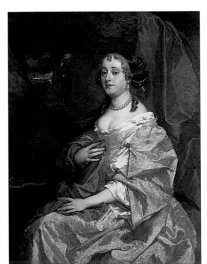

Display Breasts were a focal point of a woman's appearance during the fifteenth century when stiffened stays and bodices helped to give the appearance of high and rounded breasts.

Flat chests Fourteenth-century women wore straight, tubular bodices that completely flattened the breasts. This meant that the breasts could be hidden below the neckline of a dress, even if it was cut quite low. High, ruffled collars and wide, full skirts also drew attention away from the breasts.

Stays A fashion item from the sixteenth to the nineteenth century, stays needed help to be put on tightly. Efforts to pull them ever tighter were a source of amusement for many satirists.

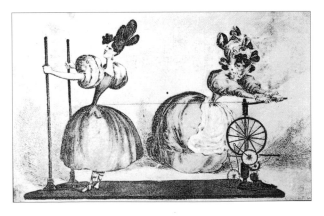

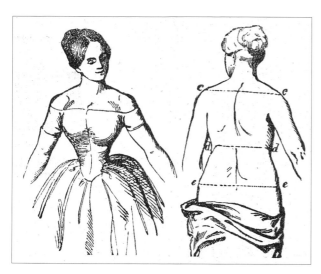

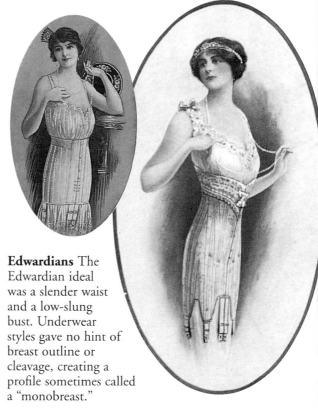

Pinched waists Corsets (above) were pulled in at the waist so tightly that they could permanently alter the waist size.

Flappers Bandeau-style bras, which were bands of elasticized material, were worn to achieve the 1920s boyish look (below).

Edwardians The Edwardian ideal was a slender waist and a low-slung bust. Underwear styles gave no hint of breast outline or cleavage, creating a profile sometimes called a "monobreast."

Early bras The first bras became popular in the late 1920s when the importance of breast support became more widely appreciated.

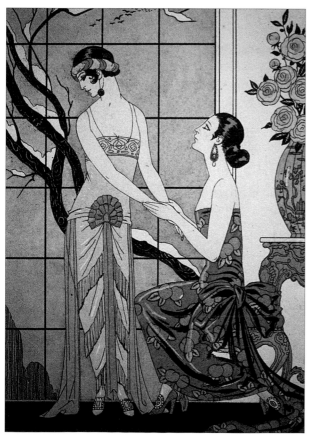

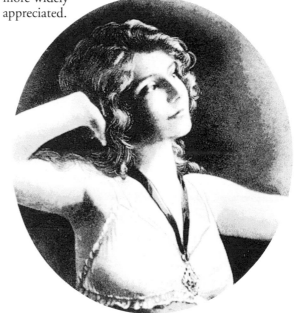

THE EMERGENCE OF THE BRA

It is thought that the word *brassiere* first appeared in American *Vogue* in 1907 and was first used in Britain in 1908; there are illustrations of brassieres, separate garments holding the breasts and suspended from shoulder straps, dating from 1913. The British magazine *The Queen* said of the brassiere in 1916 that "French and American women wear them and so must we: a *modiste* will insist on a brassière to support the figure and give it the proper up-to-date shape." The widespread adoption of the brassiere was delayed, however, by the persistence of the late Victorian and Edwardian ideal woman.

THE INTER-WAR YEARS

World War I changed all that. Women, even fashionable ones, had gained a freedom to pursue activities undreamed of by their mothers, and their clothes had to change to accommodate their new roles. Interestingly, just as the bra was coming into widespread use in the early 1920s, it veered away from supporting and rounding breasts to suppressing them almost entirely. The new woman was ideally boyish, slim, and boxy. There have been few fashions in women's clothes that so adamantly contradicted the shape of the human female as those of this period.

The 1930s saw the re-emergence of the two-breasted, rounded woman, à la Jean Harlow. Bras were something to hold rather than enhance the breast, but they had become pretty for those who could afford prettiness, being made from satins and silks and liberally trimmed with lace. The bathing beauty had been born in Hollywood, and the development of the bathing costume and the bra were to go hand in hand for a decade or so.

THE SWEATER GIRL

Lana Turner, the original "sweater girl," wore sweaters that draped her upper body fairly loosely but were tight at the waist where they ended. The front of the sweater seemed to be skewered from inside by two sharp points: Turner's breasts. Viewed from the side, her bust made a 90-degree angle with her upper body. What created this angle was the "swordpoint" bra. It had completely separate cups, each machine-sewn in a spiral of stitching that ended in the center of the cup. The cups were embedded in strong elastic, which ensured that they remained firmly in place.

When empty, a swordpoint bra retained its shape exactly, and this rigidity meant that virtually anyone could achieve the sweater-girl look. To improve the look, nothing was worn between the sweater and the bra.

FALSIES

The next innovation to delight the wearer but scandalize the nation was "falsies" – a set of pads that were worn inside the bra. Ways of enhancing the fullness of the breast were not new, but they had never been so blatant. It isn't easy to pinpoint what it was about falsies that people found so shocking.

My sister appeared wearing this sweater and we all just giggled. She'd put on about 4 inches around the bust and had gone all sort of pointy. My dad said, "You're not going out like that."

HELEN, 54, DESIGNER

Perhaps it was the notion of deception; it was all right, say, to make yourself appear taller by wearing high heels, because they were visible, and therefore no fraud was involved.

THE PUSH-UP BRA

It was a short step from the insertion of falsies into a bra to the bra that had pads built in. At first these were simply ordinary bras made from layers of material enclosing latex foam of some sort, and they totally enclosed the breast in much the same way as other bras of the period.

Then the push-up bra was born. The magic lay in the underwiring, one end of which hugged the inside edge of the cleavage while the other end lay almost in the armpit. With this kind of support anchored in shoulder straps, the smallest amount of breast tissue could be pushed upward and outward to produce what seemed to be artlessly high and natural breasts. The push-up bra was a veritable dream machine; you put it on and were invested with instant allure.

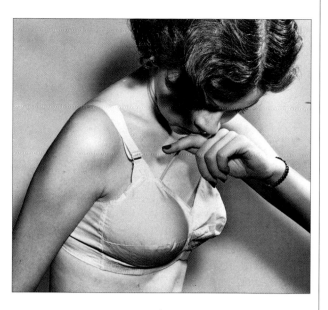

THE MERRY WIDOW

The strapless bra had always been an unsatisfactory garment. When first put on, the effect was wonderful, but no matter how ingeniously wired or how tightly fastened, it inevitably crept down the torso, taking the breast with it, and this meant that it lacked the push-up bra effect, especially after a couple of dances. In the face of this intractable problem, the underwear fashion industry came up with the merry widow. This gave the Wonderbra effect by attaching the cups to a lightly boned corset bodice, which ended a couple of inches below the waist and from which long, detachable garters hung. Nipped in at the waist, it could not slide down like the traditional strapless bra, and it gave the wearer a delicious feeling of semi-wickedness, as it closely resembled the bodices worn by the saloon girls in Hollywood westerns.

THE NEW GENERATION

The most significant changes in bra design in the last 30 years have been wrought by the development of new, man-made elastic fibers. Lighter and far stronger than rubber elastic, they are also more durable – unaffected by perspiration, body oils, deodorant, machine washing, and tumble-drying. Their strength has allowed bras to become simpler and prettier, so that the 1990s bra looks flimsy when set next to a 1950s model.

Another development has been in the range of sizes available, with the original A, B, C, D spectrum now extending from AA to HH (see p.53). Women can now choose from a huge range of bras, from the sporty to the seductive, but comfort need never be sacrificed.

Inflatable bra
This variation on the padded bra was introduced in the 1950s. Lightweight plastic containers inside the bra could be filled with air to achieve "the perfect contour" and removed when the bra was to be washed.

I'll never forget trying on my first Wonderbra in front of the mirror. The effect was stunning; I could not see my feet, let alone my waist. I thought I was a total knockout.

LOUISE, 43, LECTURER

THE WET NURSE

There is an assumption underlying contemporary debate about the relative merits of breastfeeding and bottle-feeding that we should be trying to get back to a happier time when formula milk didn't exist and all mothers breastfed their babies. The reality was not that simple. While bottle-feeding was not an option until the end of the nineteenth century, women of sufficient means could pay for their babies to be breastfed by a nursing mother of lesser status and wealth – the wet nurse. As the only means by which mothers were able to opt out of breastfeeding, the wet nurse was the feeding bottle of her day.

The practice of wet-nursing was widespread in Europe from medieval times to the end of the eighteenth century. Wherever it is found, it has to do with class. The demands of breastfeeding conflict with the perceived social duties of high-status women; the breeding potential of aristocratic women was valued more than their breastfeeding capacity, and social refinement relegated the more earthy, physical functions of motherhood to the lower orders.

ATTITUDES TOWARD WET-NURSING

In classical Greece and Rome, female domestic slaves acted as wet nurses and were not paid for their services; however, they did have better nourishment and lighter workloads than their fellow slaves. Since slaves usually lived with the family who owned them, babies were at least brought up with their parents and older siblings rather than being sent to live at the wet nurse's home, as was often the case in Europe in later periods. This willingness to part with a baby for between one and two years is in conflict with everything we now feel about the parent-child relationship.

Contemporary writings show that wet nurses were held in very low esteem by their employers in seventeenth- and eighteenth-century England, where their use was almost universal among the upper and middle classes. Elizabeth Knyve, Countess of Lincoln, a supporter of maternal breastfeeding who had 18 children and who published *The Countess of Lincoln's Nursery* in 1622, said that she had come across only two satisfactory wet nurses. She derided the notion that breastfeeding is "troublesome, noisome to one's clothes, makes one look old, endangers health," and so on.

Men seem to have been generally in favor of wet-nursing, though not without exception; the Duke of Northumberland stated categorically in 1596 that "mother's teats are best answerable to the health of a child." Certainly the evidence supports him, as it appears that babies put out to nurse had a higher rate of infant mortality than those who were not.

The medical profession by and large supported maternal breastfeeding, as did a series of Puritan writers, who believed that mothers who did not breastfeed were shirking a moral duty to their children, since Nature – and therefore, in their reasoning, God – intended it. There was the added danger that the baby might imbibe the more undesirable social characteristics of the wet nurse along with her milk.

THE NEED FOR WET NURSES

Despite constant criticisms, the use of wet nurses remained enormously popular. One clue as to how rare it was for a woman of social consequence to suckle her own children is the great pride taken by those who did in this proof of their maternal devotion. Famously, Essex Cheke, third wife of the Earl of Manchester, had recorded on her tombstone in 1658 that she had suckled seven of her children "with her own breasts." The two main factors behind the persistence of wet-nursing in Europe were probably the contraceptive property of breastfeeding (see p.94) and men's unwillingness to do without the sexual services of their wives.

WOMEN'S DUTY TO BREED

In seventeenth-century England, some 45 percent of aristocratic women died before the age of 50; about a quarter of these died from complications of childbirth. Infant mortality – variously estimated at between 118 and 158 per 1,000, allied with a significant number of deaths from disease at any age – meant that the first priority for the upper-class woman was to have as many children as she could in as short a time as possible. Only thus could those of rank hope to ensure continuity of the line and prevent their wealth and property from passing out of the family. Time spent breastfeeding was seen as time taken away from possible reproduction. The wet nurse was in this sense a fertility aid to her employer. Contrary to popular opinion, women of the poorer classes tended to have fewer children than their more elevated sisters; their children were born at longer intervals because of the prolonged periods of breastfeeding of their own and their employers' children.

HUSBANDS AGAINST MATERNAL BREASTFEEDING

There was also in Europe, as in many other parts of the world, a prohibition on sexual relations during lactation. In the case of Europe, this went back to the second-century Greek physician Galen, whose medical precepts had been accepted for some 1,500 years. He taught that "carnal copulation troubleth the blood, and so in consequence the milk." For men who could afford it, a wet nurse was a way around this state of affairs. Though wet nurses were often asked to give assurances about their sexual abstinence while suckling their charges, this was unenforceable unless they lived with their employers.

A CHANGE IN ATTITUDES

Toward the end of the eighteenth century, the practice of wet-nursing was beginning to wane in England, though it persisted in France right up to the advent of bottle-feeding at the end of the nineteenth century. In England from the 1780s onward, fashions in child-rearing, as well as in other social and educational practices, became more naturalistic and the bonds of family life became stronger. It was recognized that, in suckling their babies, mothers formed bonds with their children that were denied to them when a good part of infancy was given over to the dubious care of the wet nurse.

THE BABY, THE BREAST, AND SOCIETY

Those who study human behavior are not in total agreement about the exact significance to the infant of the breast, feeding, and nurture from the moment of birth onward. There has also been argument about whether the newborn baby has what can be called social drives – the desire to make contact with and form attachment to others. Nevertheless, there is agreement on the crucial importance of all these things in the development of the child's personality and her ability to relate to others in later life.

THE INFANT'S SOCIAL DRIVES

It used to be thought that the infant was born with virtually no other abilities than sucking and crying, but research over the last fifty years has steadily uncovered responses in very young babies that are not simply related to demanding and receiving food. In the first week of life the infant responds to the human voice differently and with more apparent pleasure than to other sounds, and particularly enjoys the sound of high-pitched voices. She can also focus on objects close to her face and shows a greater response to the human face than to other objects.

From birth the human baby shows needs for interacting with others, for being held, for being rocked, for being talked to. These needs are separate from the need to be fed, and most mothers quickly learn what their babies want depending on the cries they make.

HOW THE BABY EXPERIENCES FEEDING

The infant's early social drives are not, by themselves, as urgent as her drive for food, and they can never replace it. How food is offered is nevertheless of tremendous psychological importance. If the hungry infant is made to feel an intruder into her mother's physical and psychological space, the resulting insecurity may well remain with her into adulthood. What is so important to the young baby is that breastfeeding satisfies most of her urges at the same time. It fills her empty stomach, it gives her warmth and skin contact, and it answers her need to be touched and held and her need to touch and cling.

Bottle-fed babies can have all these experiences, but not if they are given their bottles to hold or – and it does happen, unfortunately – fed as they lie in their strollers or sit in their chairs. When the young baby puts out her hands to take her bottle, she is not making a takeover bid for it – she is reaching to touch the source of her satisfaction in the same way that a breastfed baby reaches out to touch and fondle the breast. She will enjoy holding her bottle more if she can do it while still being held by her mother.

As her life comes to include more people, sights, and sounds, the baby enjoys a wider range of pleasures, but the deep satisfaction of being lovingly fed remains of great importance to her throughout her infancy.

HOW THE BABY EXPERIENCES WEANING

Although during weaning the baby is being introduced to new tastes and sensations that she may enjoy, she is also having withdrawn from her one of the greatest pleasures of her young life – the closeness and warmth of her mother, which made being fed such a satisfying experience. The baby who is weaned abruptly or does not receive compensatory holding and cuddling during the period of weaning, whether breastfed of bottle-fed, is going to be in what can best be described as a state of shock. As well as being harmful in itself because it damages the infant's trust that what she needs will be given to her, this may lead to unhealthy attitudes toward food. The baby who refuses food during the weaning period may be making a protest about not being fed in the way she found so satisfying before.

In our culture most babies are weaned long before nature intended. The problem here has nothing to do with how the baby herself experiences weaning. She inevitably experiences weaning as a loss rather than as the gain of a more varied diet. She will experience many more losses as she grows older and will be able to sustain them better if this first loss is as gentle as possible. Weaning should be gradual, not only in the introduction of new foods but in the withdrawal of the breast.

"SPOILING" A BABY

Although it is less widespread than it used to be, there is still a school of thought that says that babies whose needs are constantly met will be "spoiled" (see p.86). The truth is that babies who usually have their needs met find the world an inviting place, where interacting with others and meeting their needs bring very satisfying responses. The baby who has had to scream for attention from day one will probably continue to do so.

If sucking on your breast is something that your baby finds satisfying even when she is not hungry, be as generous with it and with your arms, your voice, and your time as your situation allows you to be. While some people may think you're spoiling her, they won't fail to notice that she is turning into the kind of child who is always welcome.

THE INFANT SOCIAL ANIMAL

The infant will get over the loss of her mother's breast because she has no choice; whether this will help or hinder her social development will depend on how she experiences it. We are intensely social creatures, and all social life is a question of balancing the urgency of our own needs against the problems we create for ourselves if we pursue their satisfaction ruthlessly. When we've got most of what we want, it is much easier to do without what is missing and to be sympathetic to other people's needs. Long before a baby can do this for herself, her parents must do it for her by exercising control and by helping her gradually to exercise this control herself. Only by meeting the infant's deepest needs can we help a child to impose her own self-control, without which she will never be able to function happily as the social animal she is.

THE BREAST AS MODERN ICON

There can have been few periods in history when a portion of the human body has been so widely idolized as the breast has been in Western society in the latter half of the twentieth century.

THE SEXUAL BREAST

The breast has two functions: it feeds babies and it plays a large part in the sexual arousal of both men and women. Why is its second function so stressed? Why is our culture saturated by sexual images of the female breast? Why is it used to advertise products as unrelated as tires and ice cream? Although these questions seem reasonable, they are really the wrong ones. The real question is: Why is our culture so obsessed with sex? True, we need powerful sexual urges; if we didn't, the species would die out. But we would die out too if we didn't have powerful urges to eat. While there is a good deal of interest in food, as an obsession it isn't in the same league as sex. Sex is not only seen as the main conduit for rites of passage, but is felt to be the be-all and end-all of a satisfying life; so long as this is so, it is fairly predictable that the breast will remain one of our culture's most potent symbols, if only because it's the most visible sexual characteristic. As the majority of female breasts are visible even when clothed, they are a convenient focus for sexual arousal and for a large part of sexual humor and schoolboy jokes.

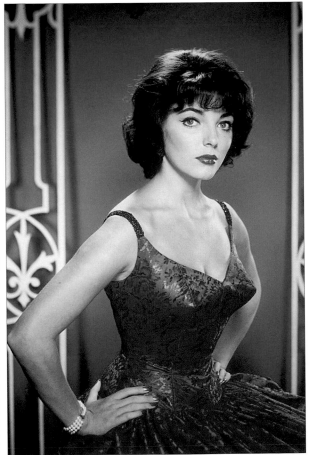

Hollywood breasts
Joan Collins is among the many Hollywood actresses to have become famous for her voluptuous looks in the 1950s.

A SOCIAL REVOLUTION

While the breast itself and people's feelings about it are obviously central to this fixation, other factors have also been at work. The last 50 years have seen the total transformation of means of communication. Images can not only be flashed around the world in no time, they can be beamed into the home, recorded, and played back at will.

The revolution that has taken place in customs and habits in the same period is no less marked. As with most revolutions, it is difficult to be certain where or when it began. In the 1940s we innocently ogled Betty Grable's legs; in the 1990s we find simulated and real sexual intercourse between naked men and women flooding into our homes via cable television. The appeal of someone like Mae West, famous for her devastating one-liners as much as for her formidable bosom, is a far cry from the panting, anonymous couples shown on the adult-movie channels.

HOLLYWOOD

Films reflect social attitudes and at the same time play a large part in forming them. It is therefore possible to trace some of the changes in attitudes toward women and their bodies by looking at films from the last 50 years or so.

Depending on your point of view, the 1950s film star Jayne Mansfield was the biggest turn-on or turn-off in the history of the breast. She typified the theory that if something is good, then more of it must be better. Her breasts threatened to overwhelm her and whoever was standing within three paces of her. She said that having babies was the sexiest thing in the world, and it is possible that her admirers felt that to be a baby and allowed to graze on the acreage of her breasts would indeed be very sexy. Her films had one purpose only – to display her bosom in a selection of dizzyingly uplifting bodices – yet she was not salacious in any way; her body did not project sex so much as play.

In one of her early 1950s films, Brigitte Bardot played a barmaid who was required to chip ice off a large block for the drink of the man who stood opposite her across the bar. Her dress was cut to within a hair's breadth of her nipples, and with each chip her bosom quivered like a live thing. Shots of these vibrations were alternated with shots of the man's face, his lips aquiver in time with her breasts. It was one of the first displays of the provocative breast in the cinema; many people were scandalized.

One of the interesting things about this scene was that Bardot's character was supposedly unaware of the effect that her breasts were having on the man across the bar. Part of the provocation lay in the implied, but not quite believable, innocence of the breast. Marilyn Monroe was more knowing, but again it was her famed vulnerability that lay at the heart of her attraction. From Bardot onward, the breasts were provocative in a way that they never had been for, say, Jean Harlow, Mae West, or Rita Hayworth. This was instantly translated into everyday life with the emphasized profile provided by the uplifting bras and the overt display of the décolleté neckline, a trend that reached its climax and died with the move to go topless.

PORNOGRAPHY

The breast is more important to soft than to hard pornography. Much hard pornography consists of close-up shots, or lingering descriptions, of variations on the sex act itself rather than the kind of foreplay that involves the breast. The big-breasted woman, however, is the image that is used everywhere to advertize pornography, and her breasts are purely sexual. This is of course distasteful to many people. For an essentially female characteristic to be the standard-bearer of what they see as perverse male sexuality is offensive.

The fact that much pornography features rampant females desperate for casual sex only offends more. The subject is complicated by the fact that blue videos for home viewing form a large part of the pornography industry, and a fair proportion of them are viewed by women as well as men. There is some debate about this: women are said to be casual and curious viewers, while men form the habitual audience.

WHEN IS PORNOGRAPHY NOT PORNOGRAPHY?

There is almost universal agreement that the plotting, characterization, acting, and cinematography of pornographic films are abysmally bad. On the other hand, one filmmaker, Russ Meyer, has an enthusiastic following of film buffs who maintain that his work is quirky, witty, and interestingly shot, and has a significance over and above the legion of improbably large-breasted women who fill it. Meyer himself freely admits that his films are expressions of his own major preoccupation – breasts.

Meyer's work illustrates the question of whether the unacceptable becomes acceptable if it is presented with enough panache and style. To his supporters, his films are hilarious spoofs of a contemporary obsession that he happens to share; to others they are just another variation of the exploitation movie. All exploitation movies draw fire on two counts: they pander to leanings that their critics feel should be suppressed, and worse, they create a market as well as cater to one. In the last analysis, in a society where women are still largely an exploited underclass – economically, sexually, and as carers for children – it is impossible to raise a cheer for even a stylish pornographer.

THE TABLOID BREAST

The essence of the attitude toward women that drives the tabloid press is that it is the breast that is desirable rather than the woman. Although the woman shown could not have rotten teeth and dandruff without anyone noticing, we are all quite clear about what she is there to display: her breasts.

When the battle lines are drawn between those who find tabloid depictions a harmless bit of fun and those who see it as the objectionable front of soft pornography, there is no common ground between the contestants. This is because pornography can be a difficult concept to grasp. What defines pornography is the reification of human beings – turning a person, or in some cases an animal, into a thing. People are sexual beings, which is to say that sexuality is a part of their essence. What pornography does is to divorce sexual characteristics from the individual person and offer them up for the arousal and satisfaction of someone else's urges. A tabloid's repeated depiction of women's breasts, aimed at the male reader, is seen by some as pornographic.

People who ridicule the campaigners against poronography are missing the point; its very existence helps to produce a climate in which women's main function is seen as servicing men's desires and is therefore a reasonable place to begin to alter this climate. It may be difficult to draw the line between the healthy contemplation of sexually exciting images and the distasteful use of a person as a sex object; but to pretend that there is no line to draw is plain silly.

FEMINISM AND THE BREAST

The battleground of the breast has had two main fronts: the attempt to wrest the breast away from the adult male and return it to the infant, and the attempt to recapture it as the sole possession of the woman. The breast was always going to pose something of a problem to the radical feminists of the

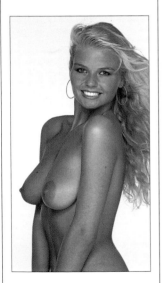

Topless models
Tabloid images of topless models are considered pornographic because they portray women as objects to excite male readers.

1960s and '70s. Predictably, and rightly, they were angered by the isolation of a single female characteristic as a focus for men's sexual fantasies without reference to the rest of a woman's body, particularly the head. In a culture where the quest for an orgasm seems to have outstripped the quest for any other holy grail, it is not strange that a fixation for the most visible sexual chacteristic has developed. Much stranger is the fact that sexual gratification has become by far the most publicly picked-over aspect of human behavior.

TWO VERSIONS OF TOPLESSNESS

One of the more bizarre episodes in the history of the battle of the sexes was the phenomenon of bra-burning: the rationale seemed to be that if men want women to have sexually desirable breasts – full, high, and pert – then women should destroy whatever helps to heighten the effect. Many women felt that the discomfort of a braless active life was too high a price for an empty gesture, however, and continued to wear their bras.

Ironically, one of the sequels to bra-burning was toplessness. Freeing themselves from being sex objects was the last thing on the minds of those who bared their breasts in the bars of San Francisco and on the beaches of the European rivieras. Of course it is possible to argue that this too was a form of liberation, that the topless breast invited inspection but no more, that its owner would select candidates for further intimacy. In the atmosphere of the time, though, this wasn't very convincing. The groups of near-naked young people holidaying nowadays on beaches and around swimming pools are much closer to that mark.

WHOSE BREAST IS IT ANYWAY?

There was no agreement in the broad feminist movement about what should be done with the breast after it had been liberated. Some women felt that it should revert to its rightful owner, the baby, while others saw the demands of breastfeeding as simply another form of tyranny, chaining women to the home and preventing them from getting out and getting on in the world at large. Interestingly, the latter view lines up people who have little in common on the same side of a social issue.

There is a strong male undercurrent of resentment toward the suckling infant (see p.84); many a man would rather bottle-feed the baby himself than see it nibbling at his partner's breast – well, his breast really. These men are not company that a bottle-feeding feminist would normally choose to keep.

As things stand now, in most of the developed Western world the bottle is more likely than the breast to be the baby's introduction to the give and take of human relationships, except among mothers of higher-than-average education (see p.87). It is hard to say precisely what effect being separated from the breast in infancy has on men's attitudes to and longings for the breast in adulthood, or women's for that matter. It is just possible that a certain kind of mastoconcupiscent (breast-loving) male chauvinist is trying to get back what he initially missed out on.

THE EXPLOITED BREAST

The breast is exploited commercially in many ways and mainly by men, who still have a near monopoly on positions at the head of business. The breast is used to manipulate the emotions of customers to make them buy products, even those that are entirely unrelated to the breast, such as cars or alcohol.

DEFINING EXPLOITATION

Book covers are an interesting example of this sort of exploitation. If the cover of a book shows a half-clad woman, this only really counts as exploitation if what is in the book has nothing to do with half-clad women. On the other hand, if the book is entirely about half-clad women, then the cover cannot really be called exploitative. A good example of the exploited breast was a paperback edition of *Oliver Twist* that showed a woman in the process of being forcibly disrobed to display a very ample bosom, and the words "He wanted more, more. He was insatiable."

Advertisements for bras are a special kind of exploitation. Although they do at least have something to do with breasts, and are directed at female buyers, they often carry the implied message that if you wear one of these, he'll be a pushover. While not directed at men, they certainly invite us to see the bra and the breasts as men would see them. More directly exploitative is the fact that these advertisements push an image of the ideal breast, suggesting that you too can have a body like this.

AN ALL-PURPOSE SELLING TOOL

What tires have to do with breasts and other parts of women's bodies may not be clear to us, but it is clear to the advertiser. Comparing one make of tires with another won't grab the average customer's attention, but if you produce calendars featuring pictures of women with bared breasts you can be sure of getting them, and your brand name, displayed in countless male-run tire shops and garages.

The implication of a good number of after-shave advertisements is that, as you're standing naked in front of the bathroom mirror splashing the stuff on, a half-naked girl will appear from nowhere to drape herself over your male body. There is at least the slimmest of connections here: many men wear after-shave to make themselves more attractive to women, and the advertisement could be a related fantasy. The beautiful girl may be out of reach, but at least you can buy the after-shave and still be part of the fantasy. The same goes for ice cream, cars, cigarettes, and a host of other "lifestyle" products.

The fact is, there does not have to be a connection, only a desire to sell a product and the knowledge that, when there isn't much difference between your product and the next, you might as well go for the feel-good factor. And what makes people feel good? Fantasized sex. And what is the sexual icon of our times? The breast. This is what is at the bottom of most advertising campaigns in which breasts are used as a selling device, and which are aimed almost exclusively at men.

THE TEENAGE BREAST

As if adolescence were not difficult enough, teenage girls have the additional worry of whether they are going to shape up to the "ideal" breast that they have seen displayed all around them since infancy. Few, if any, girls are giving serious thought to their potential lactating ability. Their concern is much more basic: are they going to develop the badge of womanliness that their culture so obviously prizes? The trend for the earlier onset of puberty over the past century means that these concerns are now affecting girls of 13 years of age or sometimes even younger.

Communal changing rooms in schools, gyms, shops, and swimming pools make it difficult for teenagers to maintain any privacy. Teenage boys, too, may be wilting over their perceived lack of potent genitalia. The breast, as always, however, being the most visible sexual characteristic, comes in for the largest share of comment. Both very small and very big breasts can be objects of amusement and derision.

AT SCHOOL

In mixed schools particularly, girls can be put under painful pressure because their development is either ahead of or behind what is thought to be the norm. Of course there is no norm; normal development takes so many forms and occurs on such differing time-scales that there are very few girls who can be described as abnormal in adolescent breast development. This may be small comfort, however, to a girl who is being teased.

Slang terms for the breast abound, but teenage boys have both the largest repertoire and the most marked preference for them: tits, jugs, jars, boobs, bouncers, Bristols, bazookas, and so on. Slang can often indicate affection or tolerance, but used by teenage boys about girls' breasts, it more often reflects a mixture of bravado, self-assertion, sexism, fear, and downright jealousy. In the early teenage years, girls' intellectual development is still ahead of that of their male classmates, and teachers frequently notice low-achieving boys teasing high-achieving girls about their breasts. Another thing teachers are aware of is the inexhaustible supply of obscene songs, in which breasts feature prominently, that boys circulate around classrooms.

MEN'S FEELINGS ABOUT WOMEN'S BREASTS

Male feelings about breasts in general are complex, and while there are common undercurrents, individual attitudes are the product of experiences both within the family and in society at large.

As children notice the similarities and differences between themselves and others, they are bound to be influenced by gender expectations. Much has been made, since Freud first put forward the theory, of penis envy in girls, though its acceptance is not as widespread as it used to be. Very little has been said about possible breast envy in boys. A brother aged three and a sister aged five were being bathed together. The boy announced to his sister, "I've got a penis. You haven't got one." His sister replied, "I know, but I've got breasts,

Adolescence for me was dreadful. My breasts seemed so big compared with everyone else's. I did everything I could to hide them. I'm still round-shouldered.

KAREN, 36,
ADMINISTRATOR

I like a woman's breasts to be just right: not too big, not too small – oh, and the areola mustn't be too big either. Saggy breasts are also a real turn-off.

ALEX, 46, ACCOUNTANT

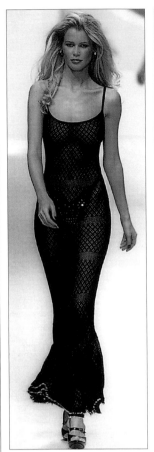

Role models
The supposedly "perfect" figures of catwalk models reflect society's view of the ideal breast, and can make the average woman feel inadequate by comparison.

> *My breasts were always big. I've only just grown into them and I'm 57! For the first time in my life I feel comfortable about my breasts. I really like them.*
SANDRA, 57, LAWYER

and when I'm grown up they're going to be big like Mommy's. And I've got *two*." End of conversation. Breasts are things that boys don't have, just as penises are things that girls don't have.

Children are profoundly affected by their parents' views and behavior. Where parents guard their nakedness or state of undress from their children as though it were shameful, it is hard for young people to feel healthily relaxed about their own or other people's bodies. If breastfeeding pointedly takes place away from children's (especially boys') eyes, they are bound to feel that it is in some way improper, and since there is nothing improper about babies, the breast is what must be kept hidden. The combination of this secret maternal breast and the flaunted breast in their culture is enough to both confuse and mislead even the best-intentioned young men.

Since the breast is seen as almost exclusively sexual in our culture, men's attitudes to it reflect their attitudes toward women and sexuality in general. Whatever their experiences in infancy and childhood, men's attitudes toward breasts are also conditioned by traditional attitudes in society that allow for men's domination, not to say ownership, of women. The amount of feeling up of their breasts to which teenage girls are subject is a direct result of these attitudes. Researchers report few cases of feeling up of penises by females.

WOMEN'S ATTITUDES TO THEIR BREASTS

A recent magazine article showed pages of photographs of breasts with no heads attached. Below each picture, the breasts' owners commented on their attitudes to their breasts. It was very cheering to find that most of the women were quite satisfied with their breasts, and some had a definite affection for them. In some cases, however, it wasn't until the unsettling adolescent years were over that the woman had been able to view her breasts objectively and discover that they were indeed all right.

We rate our breasts, as we rate nearly everything else, by comparing them with other people's. Most of the breasts on public display are highly rated by society's standards – perched high on the chest, rounded with the nipple at the center, or conical with the nipples at the point; in other words, pert. In the more down-market newspapers, heavy and even pendulous breasts are on show, frequently pushed forward into extravagant cleavages by strategically positioned arms or shoulders. Except when haute couture catwalk models wear see-through tops, boyish or very small breasts are rarely displayed. And yet many men find small breasts attractive – if indeed that is considered the final accolade. Unfortunately, the media are unlikely to point this out.

Women who have successfully breastfed their children tend to feel well satisfied with their breasts. For one thing, they have been removed from the arena where they could be rated only by whether or not they are pleasing to some man or men. The baby thought they were terrific and this gives them a status over and above any accolade they may or may not have been given as purely sexual breasts. In addition, it is hard to feel dissatisfied with anything that has done a good job well.

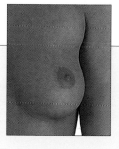

CHAPTER TWO

THE
PHYSICAL
BREAST

A woman's breasts undergo some of
the most apparent and radical
development of any part of her body.
Indeed, breasts continue to change even
after they are fully grown. A knowledge
of the anatomy and structure of your
breasts will help you to face a
lifetime of changes with confidence.

STRUCTURE OF THE BREAST

While the breasts may be of great interest to all kinds of people, to an anatomist they are of only passing interest. This is because, in anatomical terms, they are merely modified sweat glands; highly modified, it must be said, but sweat glands nonetheless – milk being the equivalent of sweat.

An anatomist would also describe the breasts as accessory reproductive organs and secondary sexual characteristics. The breasts are accessories to the main reproductive organs – the uterus, ovaries, and vagina – whose business is to conceive and produce healthy babies. This is because before artificial milk was developed, babies could not survive without breast milk. Secondary sexual characteristics are those that develop at puberty; just as deepening of the voice and the appearance of pubic hair herald fertility in men, so does the appearance of breasts in women. Emerging breasts are an outward signal of an event that would otherwise be hidden – ovulation.

With a good understanding of the workings of the breast, a woman can learn to recognize when a problem needs medical attention and, if it does, get an idea of the treatment options available to her, participate in discussions with her doctor about the possibilities, and take an active role in deciding on the ultimate line of therapy for any conditions that may arise.

ELEMENTS OF THE BREAST

Breasts have two main components: the glandular elements, comprising the lobes and ducts, and the connective tissue that forms the supporting structure. Both elements are floating in fat, which at body temperature is liquid contained in globules and accounts for most of breast volume.

The breast sits in an anatomical "pocket", formed from subcutaneous fat and skin; the chest muscles lie behind the breast. Chains of lymph nodes in the armpit pierce the upper layers of the muscles of the chest wall.

LOBES AND DUCTS

Each breast is divided into lobes, where milk is produced, and each of these contains 15–25 milk or lactiferous ducts. The lobes are pyramidal in shape and are made up of glandular tissue; each one is subdivided into lobules corresponding to the branching of the duct system. The ducts lead toward the nipple, some of them joining together on the way, and each duct widens to form a collecting sac, or lactiferous ampulla, just behind the nipple.

CONNECTIVE TISSUE

All the structures of the body are held together by connective tissue, much of it collagen; collagen is the basic material of tendons and cartilage. Within the breast, connective tissue acts as a packing material and supportive framework for all the glands; it also divides the interior of the breast into sections or septa. Just beneath the inner surface of the breast, the connective tissue is very loose and through it pass nerves, blood, and lymph vessels that supply

ANATOMY OF THE BREAST

The breasts sit outside the ribcage and the pectoral muscles. The pectoral muscles cover the chest and, when well developed, marginally influence the size of the breasts. The breasts are cushioned by a layer of fat that surrounds the glandular tissue. They merge imperceptibly with the body fat around them, except where they extend to the armpits and pierce the muscles of the chest wall.

INSIDE THE BREAST

The working parts of the breast –
that is, the glandular tissue, which
contains the lobes and the ducts – are
surrounded by fat; it is the fat that
determines the size and shape of the breast.
The proportion of glandular tissue tends to be
higher in young women, whereas in older women
the proportion of fat tends to be higher.

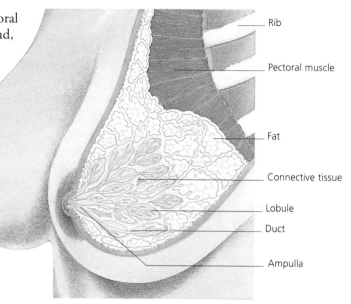

Rib
Pectoral muscle
Fat
Connective tissue
Lobule
Duct
Ampulla

POSITION ON THE MUSCLES

The inner surface of the breast lies closely
against the chest muscles, in particular the
pectoralis major but to a lesser extent the
serratus anterior and external oblique.

POSITION ON THE RIBCAGE

The breasts extend vertically
from the second to the sixth
rib, and horizontally from the
sternum across the ribcage,
with an extension into the
armpit (axillary tail).

Deltoid

Serratus
anterior

Pectoralis
major

External
oblique

Clavicle

Axillary tail
Sternum

Vertebrae

Ribs

CROSS-SECTION OF NIPPLE

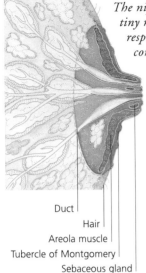

The nipple is surrounded by many tiny muscles that enable it to respond to stimulation, and contains sweat and sebaceous glands and hair follicles.

Duct
Hair
Areola muscle
Tubercle of Montgomery
Sebaceous gland

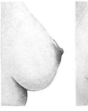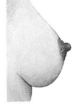

Flat nipple   Erect nipple

When the nipple's muscles contract, the areola puckers and the nipple becomes hard and elongated.

and drain the breast. Except under the nipple and the areola, the connective tissue contains liberal amounts of fat; it is this fat that is responsible for the smooth contours of the breast.

BREAST SUSPENSION

The lobes of the breast are attached to the skin by strands of connective tissue called the suspensory ligaments of Cooper; they merge with the covering of the muscles of the chest wall. These suspensory ligaments form what is in effect a sling for the breast; the sling is of a particular length and is completely inelastic. This means that, once it's stretched and the breasts sag, nothing can lift them up again except plastic surgery.

Given this once-and-for-all stretchability of the suspensory breast ligaments, it is essential that a young girl is given a good supporting bra to wear as her breasts begin to grow in size and weight, and that a woman should never go braless if she wishes to retain the pert outline of her pubertal breasts; similarly, strenuous exercise should never be undertaken without a good supportive sports bra (see p.56). During pregnancy and, most important of all, during lactation, the breasts should be well supported, and a bra worn day and night if necessary.

THE NIPPLE AND AREOLA

While the skin covering the breast is smoother, thinner, and more translucent than on most of the rest of the body, the areola's skin is even thinner and has complex sweat glands and sebaceous glands (which secrete an oily lubricating substance called sebum) and hair follicles. The surface of the areola is marked by a number of small bumps called the tubercles of Montgomery. These are sweat and sebaceous glands that become more prominent in the second half of the menstrual cycle and grow throughout pregnancy.

The nipple can be flat, round, conical, or cylindrical in shape; its color is due to the thinness and pigmentation of its skin, and it is either soft or firm according to the tone of the smooth muscle fibers found within it. These tiny muscles are quite complex: they are embedded in connective tissue and the fibers run in three different directions – around, across, and up – and extend into the connective tissue of the areola. It is these muscle fibers that make the nipple so responsive to cold or sexual arousal and make it stand out during breastfeeding so that the baby can take it in his mouth; all the fibers contract at once, and the nipple becomes firm, ridged, and elongated while the areolar skin puckers markedly. The core of the nipple is pierced by 15–25 lactiferous ducts and sinuses that open up at its tip, and it possesses many sebaceous glands that keep the nipple lubricated during breastfeeding.

IMPORTANT ANATOMICAL FEATURES

In order to get a full picture of the breast, you need to know a little more about its structure and function. It helps your understanding to be familiar with how the breast stays healthy through its blood supply and how it reacts to stimulation by way of its systems of nerves, and to be well informed about its lymphatic system in relation to breast cancer (see p.40).

> *My doctor says that it's quite normal to have lumpy breasts, but it wasn't until I saw a diagram of the breast with all its little glands inside that I really believed him.*
>
> ANNA, 26, ACCOUNTANT

BLOOD SUPPLY

Oxygen-rich blood is carried to the breast from the heart in arteries, and de-oxygenated blood returns to the heart via veins. The same major arteries that supply the chest wall also supply the breast. One artery comes from the armpit and supplies the outer half of the breast (the axillary artery); another passes from the neck down the chest and supplies the inner half of the breast (the internal mammary artery). It is the drainage of blood from the breasts through veins that has more significance, however. Malignant tumors of the breast can spread around the rest of the body by shedding cancer cells into the blood like leaves from a tree; wherever these leaves settle, a secondary breast cancer can form. The veins from the breast take blood back to the heart via those of the armpit and rib spaces, and then into veins deeper within the chest. There is even a rich network of veins that connects with the main external jugular vein and then drains almost immediately into the heart. From the heart, blood that drained from the breast circulates to the rest of the body.

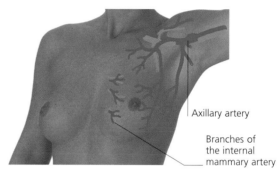

Axillary artery

Branches of the internal mammary artery

Blood supply
Oxygenated blood reaches the breast through arteries that supply the chest wall, and returns, de-oxygenated, to the heart via veins in the armpit and between the ribs.

NERVE SUPPLY

The breast has an abundant supply of nerves. The large number of sensory nerve-endings that carry signals such as touch, pain, and temperature are responsible for the exquisite sensitivity of the areola, particularly the nipple. As well as sensory nerves, the breast enjoys the bonus of extra nerves from the autonomic system – this system controls such involuntary body functions as digestion and sweating. Autonomic nerves not only control the smooth muscle fibers of the blood vessels, ducts, and nipples, but also probably form the connection whereby stimulation of the nipple can cause arousal and erection of the clitoris. This phenomenon is reported by many women – indeed, some women can achieve orgasm simply by stimulation of the nipple.

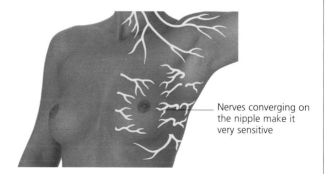

Nerves converging on the nipple make it very sensitive

Nerves
Sensory nerves in the breast carry sense signals such as touch to the brain. Autonomic nerves carry sensations from the nipple to the clitoris.

Lymph drainage of the breast

Seventy-five percent of the lymphatics in the breast drain into the lymph nodes in the armpit and from there to those above the collarbone. The lymph nodes around the breastbone receive almost all the rest.

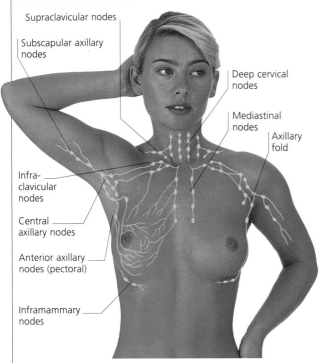

Supraclavicular nodes

Subscapular axillary nodes

Deep cervical nodes

Mediastinal nodes

Axillary fold

Infra-clavicular nodes

Central axillary nodes

Anterior axillary nodes (pectoral)

Inframammary nodes

THE LYMPHATIC SYSTEM

All organs and tissues in the body have a kind of secondary circulatory system separate from that of the blood in veins and arteries; this is called the lymphatic system. The fluid within it flows around the body and bathes individual cells and organs, like the lubricating oil of an engine. It is thin and clear, and a very pale yellow color. The lymphatic vessels are thin and membranous and very often not tubes at all but simply spaces. Lymphatic fluid drains into regional collecting points – the lymph nodes or glands. These collections of nodes filter the lymphatic fluid and attack harmful organisms, preventing most infection from passing into the bloodstream.

Regional nodes exist all over the body and will become swollen if a part draining into them is inflamed. To give a familiar example, the lymph nodes in the neck swell when there is an infection in the throat, and can be felt like a string of beads underneath the angle of the jaw.

THE BREAST'S LYMPHATIC DRAINAGE

Within the breast there is a network of lymphatic vessels (see picture above). They are found in the interlobular connective tissue and in the walls of the milk-bearing ducts. These vessels communicate with a network in the skin, especially around the nipple under the areola, and there may even be another deep submammary collection of tiny lymph vessels that lie on the surface of the chest muscles.

The lymphatic channels within the breast eventually end in the lymph nodes in the armpit (axillary lymph nodes). These lymph nodes receive and filter 75 percent of all the lymph from the breast. Of the rest, approximately 20 percent passes to the lymph nodes around the breastbone with the other 5 percent deeper into the chest. From the axillary lymph nodes, drainage goes to a group of glands called apical lymph nodes, just above the collarbone.

The lymphatic drainage of the breast is of special importance because of its relevance to the diagnosis and treatment of breast cancer; the axillary lymph nodes can be affected if a cancer spreads through the lymphatic vessels from a primary tumor in the breast. This is why feeling for lumps in the armpit and along the collarbone forms part of breast self-examination; you are not checking for tumors in these areas, but for swollen lymph nodes.

BREAST DEVELOPMENT

Though breast growth can't be seen until puberty, breast development begins very early in the embryo and can be discerned within just a few weeks of conception. Interestingly, the earliest stages are identical in male and female fetuses, so men could develop fully functioning breasts given the right hormonal conditions. After birth the breast has only two phases of development: the first at puberty with the outpouring of the hormones estrogen and progesterone; the second during pregnancy and lactation, when the milk-producing lobules become larger. If puberty is stunted or if a woman remains childless, her breasts will not develop fully.

BEFORE BIRTH

The first stage of breast development begins in the embryo at about six weeks, with a thickening in the skin called the mammary ridge or milk line. By the time the fetus is six months old, this extends from the armpit to the groin, but it soon dies back, leaving two breast buds on the upper half of the chest.

Occasionally, rudimentary mammary glands develop along the milk line forming additional nipples or breasts that sometimes persist into adult life (see p.45). More rarely, the two breast buds fade away with the rest of the milk line, so that the nipples are absent from birth. Because the initial development of the milk line is the same in male and female fetuses, both of these quirks of development can occur in men as well as women. Extra nipples and breasts or absent nipples can be corrected only with cosmetic surgery.

When a female fetus is about six months old, 15–20 solid columns of cells grow inward from each breast bud. Each column becomes a separate "sweat" or exocrine gland, with its own separate duct leading to the nipple. By about the eighth or ninth month of fetal development, these columns of cells have become hollow so that, by birth, a nipple and a rudimentary milk-duct system have formed. No further development takes place until puberty.

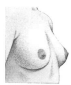

The milk line
Running from the armpit down to the groin, the milk line is the most common site of extra nipples.

ADOLESCENCE

The first external signs of breast development appear at the age of 10 or 11, though it can be as late as 14. The ovaries start to secrete estrogen, leading to an accumulation of fat in the connective tissue that causes the breasts to enlarge.

The duct system also begins to develop, but only to the point of forming cellular knobs at the end of the ducts. As far as we know, the mechanism that secretes milk doesn't develop until pregnancy.

The onset of breast changes is rapidly followed by other outward signs of puberty, including the appearance of pubic hair and armpit hair.

STAGES OF DEVELOPMENT

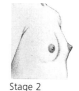
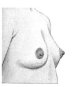

Stage 1   Stage 2   Stage 3   Stage 4

1 Before puberty
The breast is flat except for the nipple, which projects from the areola.

2 Development begins
The areola becomes a prominent bud.

3 Growth of breast tissue
Fat and glandular tissue within the breasts increase.

4 The adolescent breast
With further development, the areola flattens over the breast tissue.

Although the breasts may appear fully grown within a few years of puberty, strictly speaking their development is not complete until they have fulfilled their biological function – that is, until a woman carries a pregnancy to term and breastfeeds her baby, when they will undergo further changes.

MATURITY OF THE BREAST

Once a girl reaches puberty, and ovulation and the menstrual cycle begin, the breasts start to mature, forming real secretory glands at the ends of the milk ducts. Initially these glands are very primitive and may consist of only one or two layers of cells surrounded by a base membrane. Between this membrane and the glandular cells are cells of another type, called myoepithelial cells. These myoepithelial cells are the ones that contract and squeeze milk from the gland if pregnancy occurs and milk production takes place.

With further growth, the lobes of the glands become separated from one another by dense connective tissue and fat deposits. This tissue is easily stretched and allows the enlargement that occurs during pregnancy when the glandular elements swell and grow. The duct system grows considerably after conception, and many more glands and lobules are formed. This causes the breast to increase in size as it matures to fulfil its role of providing food for a baby.

CYCLICAL BREAST CHANGES

Every month a fertile woman experiences fluctuations in hormone levels as part of the menstrual cycle. These hormones can cause breast tenderness and even pain prior to menstruation.

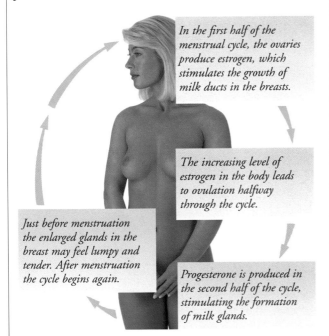

In the first half of the menstrual cycle, the ovaries produce estrogen, which stimulates the growth of milk ducts in the breasts.

The increasing level of estrogen in the body leads to ovulation halfway through the cycle.

Just before menstruation the enlarged glands in the breast may feel lumpy and tender. After menstruation the cycle begins again.

Progesterone is produced in the second half of the cycle, stimulating the formation of milk glands.

CYCLICAL CHANGE

Most women notice that just before menstruation their breasts enlarge and their nipples become sensitive and even painful. The texture of the breasts changes and they can become rather lumpy, with small discrete swellings that resemble orange pits in both texture and size. These lumps are glands in the breast that enlarge in preparation for pregnancy. If pregnancy doesn't occur, they return to normal size and become imperceptible to the touch within a few days, ready for regrowth the next month. These changes in the breast are only one part of many changes that occur in the female body as the result of the monthly ebb and flow of the female hormones estrogen and progesterone.

THE AGING BREAST

As we get older, our breasts tend to sag and flatten; the larger the breasts, the more they sag. With menopause comes a reduction in stimulation by the hormone estrogen to all tissues of the body, including breast tissue; this results in a reduction in the glandular tissue of the breasts, so they lose their earlier fullness. Much of the connective tissue in the breast is composed of a fibrous protein called collagen, which needs estrogen to keep it healthy. Without estrogen, it becomes dehydrated and inelastic. Once the collagen has lost its shape and stretchability, it cannot return to its former state.

In some women menopause can bring with it an enormous increase in the size of the breasts. A possible explanation for this is the increase with age of anovulatory cycles (cycles in which we don't ovulate). In anovulatory cycles there is no progesterone to control the effect of estrogen and no cutoff. The breasts are therefore exposed to prolonged periods of unopposed estrogen stimulation and swell as a result. The action of unopposed estrogen on the breasts also leads to swelling of the remaining glands in the breast and an increase in fat cells. As a result the breasts may be tender and even painful (mastalgia) at menopause. Decreasing caffeine relieves mastalgia for some women, but the condition is temporary and not associated with malignancy.

DEVELOPMENT AND BENIGN BREAST CHANGE

As the various components of the breast continue to develop over the years, changes take place in all the tissues, which can give rise to lumps, cysts, and sometimes nipple discharge. At one time these changes were thought of as diseases. We no longer see them even as abnormal but simply as variations or aberrations of normal that are benign and require no treatment (see p.120).

HORMONES AND THE BREAST

The breast contains millions of receptor cells, which respond to hormones. At puberty, a girl's breasts change in size and shape under the influence of the hormones that govern menstruation – estrogen and progesterone. Sensitivity to these hormones varies from one woman to the next and determines the ultimate size of the breasts. The more sensitive the hormone receptors are, the larger the breasts will become (see p.46).

Throughout a woman's fertile years the breasts are influenced by the hormones that control the menstrual cycle (see left). This hormonal activity causes changes inside the breasts, which is why some women experience premenstrual breast tenderness or pain. The same cycle of waxing and waning continues throughout fertile life, exposing the breasts to regular surges of estrogen, except when a woman is either pregnant or breastfeeding. The earlier menstruation starts and the later the menopause, the fewer the pregnancies and the less the breastfeeding, then the more estrogen a woman is exposed to during her lifetime. This exposure may be related to cancer risk (see p.143).

During pregnancy, breast tissue springs to life under the influence of the hormone called human placental lactogen (HPL); milk production is ruled by two other powerful hormones, namely prolactin and oxytocin, with further contributions from growth hormone and thyroid hormone (see p.147).

As ovarian function wanes in middle age, so does the ripeness of the breasts. Unless the ovarian hormones are replaced with some form of hormone replacement therapy, the breasts will lose their fullness and elasticity.

SIZE AND SHAPE

"May your breasts stay high and round like a young girl's." It could almost be a mother's prayer for her daughter, or a bra manufacturer's promise to a prospective customer. It is actually a traditional curse from Papua New Guinea and highlights the ethnic and cultural differences in attitudes to the breast. Girlish breasts on a mature woman would indicate childlessness, and in Papua New Guinea that would indeed be seen as a curse.

Nevertheless, the structure of the breast is the same the world over in relation to its primary function – lactation. The great variety that we see stems from the assortment of shapes and sizes of the layer of subcutaneous fat on which the nipple sits. This variation is not related to race or ethnic group; there are more differences within races than between races. The three body types to which all human beings roughly conform – endomorphic (fat or heavy), mesomorphic (muscular and athletic), and ectomorphic (thin and light) – are found in all races, though there may be regional clustering of particular types. A woman's physical type does not determine the volume and shape of her breasts; each type shows the whole range of variation from scant and boyish to large and pendulous.

WHAT IS NORMAL?

The images of the breast touted by the fashion and advertising industries fall within such narrow limits – pert, rounded, firm, and hairless – that it is not surprising that many women feel their breasts are not "normal." The fact is that all breasts are capable of producing milk, and as such they are normal, though they come in a huge variety of shapes and sizes.

Every breast, however, regardless of size or shape, has a nipple surrounded by a disc-shaped area, the areola, which is a darker color than the skin surrounding it. The size and shape of mature women's breasts vary greatly among individuals and can even vary in individual women, particularly during pregnancy and lactation and at various times in the menstrual cycle.

SOME COMMON VARIATIONS

Some women think their breasts are abnormal not just because of their shape, but also their size. Other variations are usually due to quirks of development, but are still common enough to be regarded as normal and entirely harmless.

HAIRS ON THE NIPPLE

There's hardly a woman who doesn't have at least one hair on her breasts, usually around the areola, and some women have many. While their presence is normal they can be a cause of embarrassment, especially if they are coarse and dark, and some women have them permanently removed by electrolysis. For others, occasional shaving or plucking or the use of a depilatory cream is enough. After menopause, the hair around the breasts grows more slowly and may eventually disappear with age.

INVERTED NIPPLES

The nipple has two forms – everted (turning outward) and inverted (turning inward). Inverted nipples are quite common and are simply a variation of the norm, though they can be a cause of great concern for women whose nipples take up this conformation. They occur because the lactiferous ducts that tether the nipple are too short. Gentle, sustained suction stretches the ducts and allows the nipple to come "out." Suction devices such as nipple shells are widely available. A common worry is that breastfeeding will not be possible, but in fact the use of a breast shell can often solve this problem. It is possible to have cosmetic surgery to correct an inverted nipple (see p.107), but as the milk ducts are often cut across, this will definitely make breastfeeding an impossibility afterward. A previously everted nipple may become inverted as the result of nipple disease (see p.132).

ACCESSORY NIPPLES

The breasts develop from a mammary ridge or milk line (see p.41) that runs from the upper chest to the groin, and it is possible for an extra nipple to develop along this strand of breast tissue in the fetus – rarely with an underlying breast. This is known as polymastia, and, though it is more commonly found in women, it can happen in men too. The extra nipple often looks like a mole, so the woman doesn't realize what it is, but it may lactate at the same time as the "real" breasts and cause embarrassment. This extra nipple and breast is not in any way abnormal and should not be a cause for concern, given its embryonic origins. Nonetheless, its removal before puberty is an option to be considered if it is very prominent and likely to become a source of further embarrassment during the self-conscious teenage years.

ASYMMETRY

It is very rare indeed for a woman's breasts to be entirely symmetrical; one is usually larger and consequently may be heavier and sit lower than the other. The difference between the right and left breast is rarely very great, but occasionally it is obvious to the degree that a different cup-size may be needed for each breast. One friend of mine used to buy two bras in different sizes, one to accommodate her small breast and a larger one to accommodate her bigger breast. She'd cut them in half and sew the odd halves together – a quite unsatisfactory arrangement. Having bras especially made is prohibitively expensive. For some women, having asymmetrical breasts is of no concern, but for others it is disconcerting and, if desired, can be corrected with plastic surgery (see p.107), either by enlarging one breast or by reducing the other.

THE TINY OR FLAT BREAST

Breasts come in all shapes and sizes, and even the most minuscule, though sometimes disappointing to the individual, is nonetheless normal and fully capable of breastfeeding a baby. While you may not be so generously endowed as some of your sisters, rest assured that nature has not sold you out in the

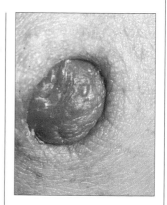

Inverted nipples
Inward-turning nipples are quite common. They are of concern only if the inversion is sudden, which may indicate breast disease.

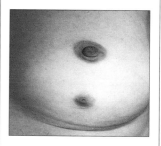

Supernumerary nipples
Some people are born with extra nipples. These rarely have separate breast tissue, but where they do they function as normal breasts.

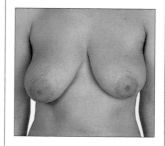

Asymmetry
It is very rare for a woman to have identical breasts, but where the difference in breast size is particularly noticeable the breasts are said to be asymmetrical.

lactation stakes. You may find that during pregnancy and lactation your breasts fill out to what you feel are satisfying proportions. The breasts of anorexia nervosa sufferers shrink to their pre-pubertal size due, at least in part, to lack of hormone stimulation. Any condition that prevents ovulation and arrests menstruation, such as overtraining in women athletes or anorexia, will result in shriveling of the breasts. Large pectoral muscles, like those of female body-builders, should not be mistaken for the soft, rounded, real thing.

LARGE BREASTS

The development of breasts at puberty (see p.41) is dependent on the sensitivity of breast tissue to the secretion of estrogen, which can vary among women. Sometimes breast tissue can be hypersensitive to small amounts of estrogen, and the breasts enlarge and become heavy very rapidly, even making stretch marks in the skin. This uncontrolled overgrowth of the breasts in pubescent girls is called juvenile or virginal hypertrophy. If unsupported, the suspensory ligaments of Cooper that hold the breasts (see p.38) will become overstretched and the breasts will sag. Even with good support, very heavy breasts can become pendulous.

For a teenager, breasts of this size and shape can be very embarrassing; added to this is the difficulty of finding large bras and clothes that will accommodate them, plus the discomfort to the shoulders as the bra straps take the strain of the weight. Many girls with large breasts develop a stoop in an attempt to camouflage their size, and may suffer from backache and neckache as a result. Negotiating the teenage years can be difficult in itself without having to cope with extremely large breasts, and in my opinion all girls with this problem should be informed of the possibility of surgical breast reduction (see p.110) and offered counseling. The results of such operations are usually very good.

Older men
Most men over seventy have obvious breasts. Due to decreasing levels of testosterone, estrogen once again dominates the hormonal balance, often resulting in breast growth.

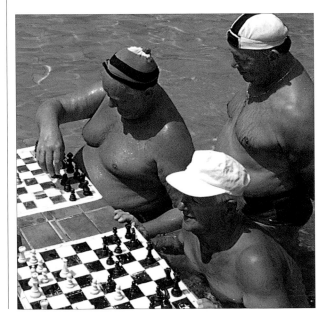

Moving the nipple and areolar skin, however, may affect the ability to breastfeed, though this depends on the surgical technique used – ask your surgeon about operations that can preserve the milk ducts.

BREASTS IN MEN

Men's breasts appear rudimentary when compared with female breasts, but have basically the same structure. Every man has breast tissue and the male nipple is identical to its female counterpart; it is equally sensitive and erogenous. At the end of a man's fertile life, as the activity of the testes wanes, breasts almost universally make an appearance.

Breast development in boys (gynecomastia) can occur in early puberty. Unpredictable hormone secretion at this time may mean that androgen (the male hormone) production temporarily lags behind that of estrogen, and tiny breasts may appear.

KNOW YOUR BREASTS

Just as you learn about your hair type and skin type in order to care for your hair and skin, so it makes sense to learn about your breasts. This is important because it's by noticing changes when you carry out breast self-examination (see pp.58–63) that you can take prompt action to investigate any problems.

YOUR BREASTS THROUGH LIFE

Your breasts are going to go through normal changes throughout your life in very much the same way as other organs in your body. They will also age, and in this context I don't mean that they will flatten or sag. I mean that the elements within them will bud, flower, and wither.

All the glandular components will wax and wane in this way, but they don't necessarily do so to the same timetable. The growth cycle of the lobules occurs first, followed by that of the glands, and lastly the ducts. Lobular development happens mostly in the late teens and early 20s and shows up as the large number of fibroadenomas (see p.129) in this age group. Tender, lumpy breasts and mastalgia, caused by menstrual hormones (see pp.122–24), are mainly a feature of our 30s, although they can also occur earlier and later. The duct development cycle occurs in our 40s and 50s. In post-menopausal women ectasia, or dilation of the ducts (see p.132), may give rise to benign conditions such as nipple discharge and nipple inversion.

These phases of development are not completely distinct but overlap so that a woman may, for example, experience pre-menstrual breast pain in her 40s even while the ducts in her breasts are beginning to dilate.

YOUR BREASTS AND YOUR LIFESTYLE

We are all living in a soup of environmental factors that may affect the health of our breasts. The Western diet, for instance, is often quoted as increasing the risk of breast cancer (see p.148), the culprits being animal fats and red meat. There is nowhere near enough evidence, however, to advise all women to cut down on these valuable foodstuffs. Obesity may be a mild risk factor for breast cancer. Alcohol, too, is said to play a part (see p.149), but I'm sure we can all go on drinking moderately without increasing our odds of getting breast cancer. Smoking, on the other hand, seems to be a mitigating factor (see p.149) – but who would dream of taking up cigarettes to reduce the risk of contracting cancer of the breast? On the downside, smoking is clearly linked to nipple infections and some of their less pleasant complications (see p.135). Taking hormones in the form of the combined oral contraceptive pill or HRT (see pp.145–46) may increase your chances of breast cancer, but if it does it's in the tiniest amount. Another effect of the pill, noticed by many women, is a slight increase in the size of the breasts.

Eating a balanced diet and getting regular exercise – including pectoral exercises to firm up your chest muscles – are the basic prerequisites for good breast health, but in the end we're all probably the creatures of our genes.

While changes in genes (mutations, see p.142) can promote cancer, they occur rarely, and one gene change on its own is almost surely not enough. Since 15 percent of cancer risk appears to relate to lifestyle, interactions between our lifestyle and our genes slightly increase our susceptibility to breast cancer.

YOUR BREAST TYPE

No two breasts are the same, not even on the same woman. Some women have naturally "lumpy" breasts, which can make it difficult to identify a new lump if one appears. Some breasts are more fibrous than others, and the large areas of fibrous tissue show up on mammography as cloudy and whitish – doctors describe such breasts as dense.

As we age our breasts become less dense (see below), but we all vary. In 1976, an American radiologist named John Wolfe drew up a classification system for breasts based on density. He identified four types, distinguished by the relative proportions of fat and glandular tissue. Your Wolfe type is as individual to you as your skin type or your hair color.

BREAST DENSITY AND AGE

As a general rule, the younger you are the more dense your breasts, and this is one of the reasons why mammography (see pp.64–65) is not useful for screening young or pre-menstrual women. HRT can stall the ageing process of the breasts so that on a mammogram post-menopausal breasts can look younger. Abnormal shadows are notoriously difficult to spot on mammograms of dense breasts, so other screening methods such as ultrasound (see p.68) are used in young women at high risk for breast cancer.

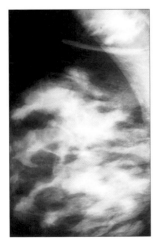

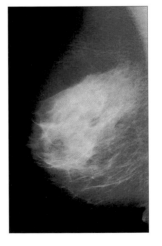

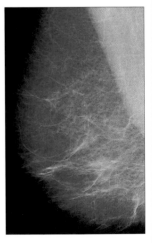

UNDER 30
On this mammogram of a young breast, the active glandular tissue appears as a white area occupying almost the entire image.

30 TO 40
The glandular tissue is still dominant, but there is an increase in fatty tissue, which shows up as darker areas around the white.

MID-40s
As menopause approaches, the glandular tissue continues to reduce, so abnormalities are easier to detect on a mammogram.

OVER 55
The glandular tissue, now much reduced, appears as a fine network over the darker areas of fatty tissue.

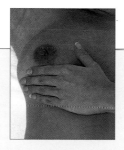

CHAPTER THREE

BREAST CARE

The health of your breasts is in your
hands, from finding a well-fitting bra
to making sure that regular examinations
are carried out. It is vital for your
physical health and emotional well-being
that you take on this responsibility.
Learning how to care for your breasts
will help you maintain their health all
through your life.

EVERYDAY BREAST CARE

The breasts don't need much in the way of beauty routines, but they do need to be treated with care, since their skin is very delicate. While many "beauty" treatments for the breasts exist, these generally are entirely worthless.

SKIN CARE

The skin of the breasts, particularly over the areola and the nipple, is thinner and more translucent than elsewhere on the body because the lower layers contain less collagen. This delicate skin needs to be treated gently, and should never be subjected to scrubbing or rough toweling, as this can make the nipples sore and tender, particularly in the week prior to menstruation. The nipple and areola may become dry and flake premenstrually, so it's a good idea to moisturize them twice a week with an unperfumed moisturizer.

Eczema can occur on the nipples. Should you get a persistent patch, consult your doctor for a precise diagnosis and specific treatment, as in rare cases it can be a symptom of a more serious condition called Paget's disease (see p.136).

SUN PROTECTION

The breasts of white-skinned women can very easily become sunburned, because the chest skin contains few melanocytes – cells that protect the skin from sunburn by producing the tanning pigment melanin. Until a tan is well established, you should apply a sun block with a sun protection factor (SPF) greater than 15 every two hours or so, and after swimming.

A gentle breaking-in period will help the skin accommodate the bright UV rays: no more than five minutes' exposure on the first day, no more than ten minutes on the second, and an additional five minutes on each succeeding day, up to half an hour. Even after this regime you may be sunburned if you expose your breasts to sun for longer than two hours before they're given the opportunity to tan slowly.

CAN BEAUTY REGIMES HELP THE BREASTS?

When I was a girl, the favorite technique among my friends for keeping your breasts pert was to bathe them first with hot water and then with cold water. This puckered up the areola and made the nipple erect, which was perhaps taken as a sign of uplift. It only represented a change in the slackness of the skin, however, and a transient one at that.

All kinds of beauty products are peddled in the hope of convincing women that potions, lotions, and creams rubbed into the skin will help them keep the shape of their breasts or even increase their size. In fact the only way to maintain the shape of the breasts is by the early wearing of bras (see p.52). Nothing applied to the skin can alter their shape or consistency, both of which are determined by your own individual response to estrogens secreted during puberty, and thereafter with each menstrual cycle. Your breasts can be changed only from the inside, by the hormones manufactured inside your body.

BREAST EXERCISES

Exercises won't actually change the shape or size of your breasts. What you can do with exercise is strengthen and tone your pectoral muscles. Given that the suspensory ligaments that support the breasts are attached to the pectoral muscle, it's conceivable – just – that exercises to tone this muscle could lift the breasts perhaps ½ inch (1 centimeter) or thicken the pad of muscle on which the breast sits, thereby increasing your bust measurement by perhaps ¾ inch (2 centimeters). If you're interested in increments of this order, then try the following exercises.

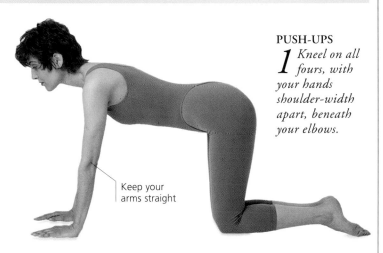

PUSH-UPS

1 Kneel on all fours, with your hands shoulder-width apart, beneath your elbows.

Keep your arms straight

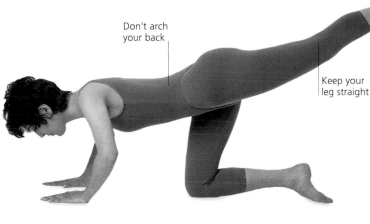

Don't arch your back

Keep your leg straight

2 Stretch your left leg out behind you with your toes pointing back. Bend your elbows to lower your chest nearly to the floor, keeping your shoulders in line with your hands. Repeat this several times, then repeat the whole sequence with your right leg out behind.

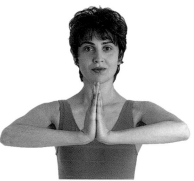

PALM PRESSES

Press your palms together in front of your breasts. Hold for five seconds, relax, and repeat ten times.

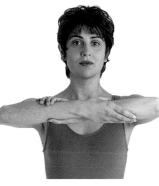

FOREARM GRIP

Grasp your forearms at shoulder level and pull without letting go. Repeat ten times.

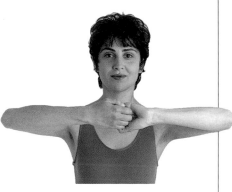

FINGER LOCK

Curl your fingers, lock them together at shoulder height, and pull. Hold for five seconds. Repeat ten times.

BRAS

Wearing a bra is one of the best things you can do for your breasts. A bra that's been chosen with care and fits well can make you more comfortable, enhance your appearance, and in the long term help keep your breasts from sagging.

WHO NEEDS A BRA?

Depending on their sensitivity to estrogen, a girl's breasts can grow quite big very quickly during the adolescent years, producing silvery stretch marks on the skin and stretching suspensory ligaments that will ultimately result in sagging. Once these ligaments lose their tightness, it can never be regained. Precautions, in the form of a bra, have to be taken sooner rather than later.

A criterion for bra-wearing when I was a girl was to see if the crease under the breasts was deep enough to hold a pencil. In fact, this wouldn't happen until the breasts were already a B cup, which is leaving it go too long. As soon as there's any weight in the breasts it's the time to start wearing a bra.

Adolescent girls are often shy about their breasts and can find the sudden appearance of two bumps at the front of the chest, which interfere with sports, an embarrassment. Mothers can help by forewarning their daughters about

ELEMENTS OF THE BRA

Whatever style of bra you choose, it should have adjustable straps and hooks and should give good support, either with strong elastic or underwiring.

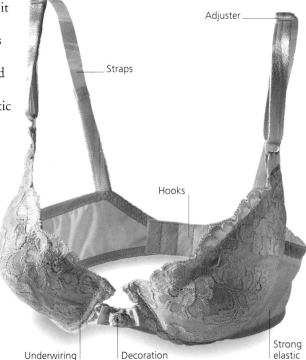

Adjuster

Straps

Hooks

Underwiring | Decoration | Strong elastic

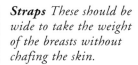

Straps *These should be wide to take the weight of the breasts without chafing the skin.*

Adjusters *These allow the straps to be adjusted to fit well on the shoulders.*

Hooks *Two or three sets of eyes allow you to adjust the bra's width across your back.*

Underwiring *Wire stitched into seams beneath the cups gives strong support.*

Padding *A bra may come with interior padding or a set of removable pads.*

MEASURING UP

*1 Always wear a bra when measuring your bra size. Measure around your rib cage just under your breasts as shown below. Add 5 inches to an odd number or 4 to an even number to get your bra back size (see **Back size** table, right).*

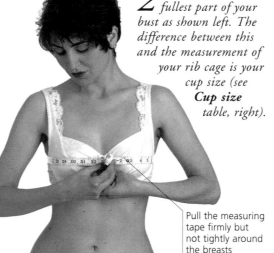

2 Loosely measure the fullest part of your bust as shown left. The difference between this and the measurement of your rib cage is your cup size (see **Cup size** *table, right).*

Pull the measuring tape firmly but not tightly around the breasts

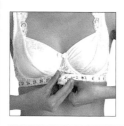

BACK SIZE		CUP SIZE	
Rib cage	Bra back size	Difference in inches	Cup size
25-26	30	5	A
27-28	32	6	B
29-30	34	7	C
31-32	36	8	D
33-34	38	9	DD
35-36	40	10	E
37-38	42	11	F
39-40	44	12	FF
41-42	46	13	G
43-44	48	14	GG
45-46	50	15	H

breast development and encouraging them to see the acquisition of breasts as a rite of passage to adulthood that is to be treasured. The whole subject of bras can be embarrassing too, but a teenage girl has every right to feel comfortable with her first bra and should be introduced to the notion of wearing one long before she needs it. Many teenagers are eager to wear a bra, especially if their friends at school have started wearing theirs.

Any sport that results in a jogging movement will mean that the suspensory ligaments take the weight of the breast every few seconds. A sporty adolescent therefore needs breast support even earlier than her less active sisters.

FINDING THE RIGHT BRA

Most of us don't seek expert advice when buying a bra. We go on buying the same-size bra for years without considering whether it still fits. We even fall into the trap of buying without trying. As a result, the bra rarely fits well or gives support where it's needed. It is estimated that about 80 percent of women are wearing the wrong size bra. This is a great pity, because an ill-fitting bra not only feels uncomfortable when you're wearing it but can also cause aches and pains in the long run. What's more, even the most expensive designer clothes won't look good if you're wearing a lumpy, poorly fitting bra underneath. Get a new one, though, and have it fitted properly, and even your old T-shirt will look better.

You'll stand a better chance of being satisfied with your next purchase if you measure properly first and try several bras to find one that really fits. You can measure yourself, but you'll find it easier and more accurate if a friend or your partner helps you. Best of all, have a fitting at a specialist lingerie shop or at the lingerie department of a large department store; there's no charge for this service and it can be a revelation – not just in terms of your size but also of the comfort and shape a bra can give.

BACK AND CUP PROBLEMS

A common mistake is to change to a bra in a larger back size when what is really needed is a bigger cup size. Your back size is largely determined by your rib cage, so it's unlikely to change once you reach adulthood. A woman who wears a size 34B and feels she needs a larger bra is likely to go out and buy a 36B, when in fact what she needs is a 34C. This is a particular problem for very large-breasted women: a woman who needs, say, a 34H but can't find an H-cup bra may end up buying a 42DD to obtain the right cup size. Since the back size is too large, however, the bra will not give her the support she needs.

CHOOSING A BRA

It is important to fit your bra properly to avoid "bra-strap back," a fairly common complaint caused by large breasts and ill-fitting bras. One estimate has it that two-thirds of large-breasted women suffer from pain between the shoulder blades and at the base of the neck, made worse by wearing the wrong bra and poor posture. It is unfortunate that large-breasted women, who have

PUTTING ON A BRA

1 Slip the bra straps over your shoulders and, as you pull the ends together to fasten them, lean forward so that your breasts fall into the cups. Fasten the bra.

2 Slide your left hand inside the right cup under your breast, and scoop it upward so that it is not flattened against the chest wall by the bra. Repeat for the other breast.

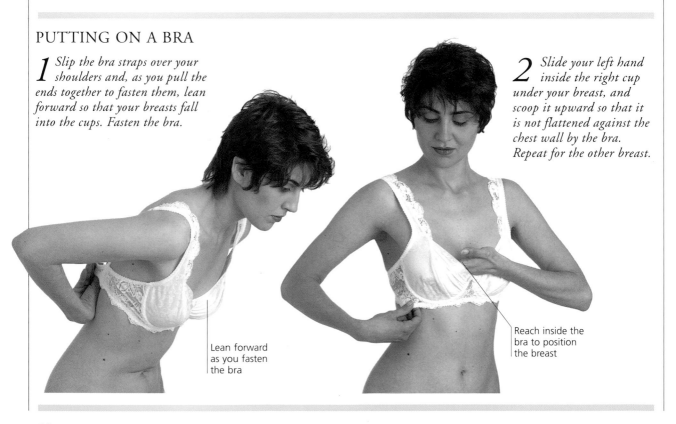

Lean forward as you fasten the bra

Reach inside the bra to position the breast

most to gain from wearing a well-fitted bra, are often too self-conscious to have a proper fitting, and that many women are unaware of the wide range of sizes and styles available on the market.

Getting the right size is only the first step; there are some other features to check before settling on a bra. Your personal preferences and the look you are trying to achieve must also be taken into consideration – do you prefer front or back fastenings, for instance, and do you want to make the most of your breasts or play them down? You must try on a bra and scrutinize it closely to get the best result. If you're buying a bra to wear under a special outfit, bring the outfit with you so you can be sure of getting what you need, especially for clothes that are cut very low in the front or back.

Not all bras of the same size fit the same way. Sometimes a different style rather than a different size may produce the effect you want. An underwired bra rather than one with wider straps may be a better choice if you need more support; straps that cut into the shoulder signal that this is the case. Similarly, a push-up bra may produce better cleavage than one that pushes the breasts out to the sides. (For a range of bra styles, see p.56.) Finally, don't be too rigid about your bra size. All clothing sizes can vary between manufacturers, and a 38D in one brand could easily be a 36C in another.

Does it fit?
When you try on a bra, scrutinize it closely to see if there are any aspects of the fit that could be improved.

If the straps cut into your shoulder, you may need wider straps or underwiring

If the breasts bulge along the top of the cups, the cups are too small or too pointed

Check the bra sides for any seams that interfere with the profile

For a clean cleavage, the bra must lift and separate the breasts

Metal adjusters near the shoulder will cut into the skin

Lace-trimmed straps can irritate the shoulders if your breasts are heavy

Bulges at the armpits mean the bra back size is too small or the side panels too narrow

If the bra pushes your breasts out to the side, it will widen your front-facing outline

TYPES OF BRAS

There is a huge range of bras available. Some – such as nursing bras – are designed for special situations; others are intended to suit different sizes of breasts or styles of clothes. Try various types to obtain different effects.

SPECIAL SITUATIONS

Nursing bra Milk-filled breasts are heavy, so a nursing bra needs broad, non-slip straps. The cups unfasten with a zip or a hook on the strap.

A zip front is best for larger sizes

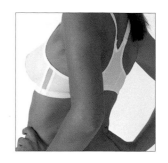

Sports bra The straps are set close together so they don't slip off the shoulders, and a broad band below the breasts stops it riding up.

FLATTERING YOUR FIGURE

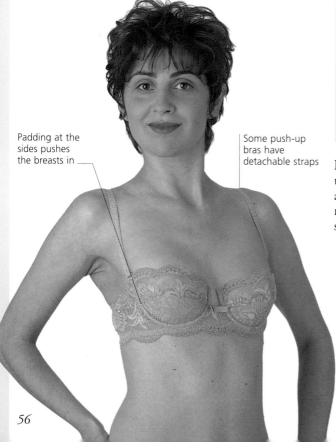

Padding at the sides pushes the breasts in

Some push-up bras have detachable straps

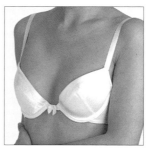

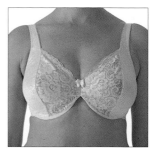

Push-up bra Padding underneath the breasts and strong support makes the most of small breasts.

Minimizer bra Popular with large-breasted women, this pushes the breasts out to the sides rather than the front.

Push-in bra A combination of padding and clever design maximizes the breasts and creates or emphasizes a cleavage. The push-in is most suitable for smaller breasts as large breasts tend to bulge over the cups, creating a visible line.

SPECIAL CLOTHES

Long-line bra Backless and strapless, a long-line bra will work under most evening dresses. The suspenders are optional, but they do help to keep the bra from riding up by anchoring it to your stockings.

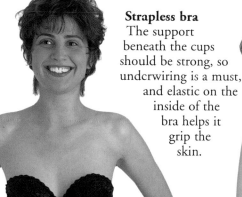

Strapless bra The support beneath the cups should be strong, so underwiring is a must, and elastic on the inside of the bra helps it grip the skin.

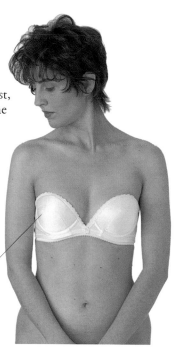

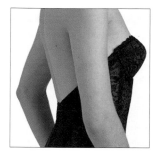

A boned bodice keeps the bra in place

Stiffened fabric for the cups gives extra support

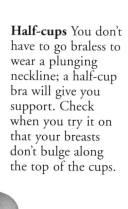

Half-cups You don't have to go braless to wear a plunging neckline; a half-cup bra will give you support. Check when you try it on that your breasts don't bulge along the top of the cups.

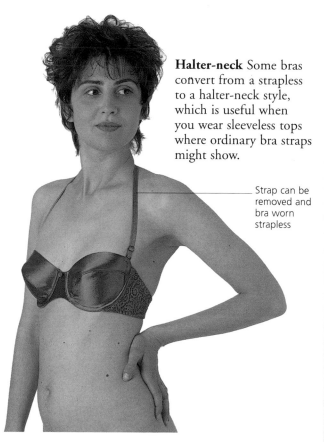

Halter-neck Some bras convert from a strapless to a halter-neck style, which is useful when you wear sleeveless tops where ordinary bra straps might show.

Strap can be removed and bra worn strapless

Underwiring is essential with low-cut cups

BREAST SELF-EXAMINATION

Most women who examine their breasts regularly will never find a lump, let alone a malignant one. Breast self-examination (BSE) is simply a way to explore your body, become familiar with it, and learn to be proud of it. You don't have to feel that you're looking for anything in particular; you're simply getting to know what your breasts usually feel like so that you can recognize something unusual should it appear.

Every woman should start doing BSE in the teenage years as soon as she develops breasts and keep on doing it until she dies. There should be no time in your life when you stop or interrupt this routine.

WOMEN WHO DO

Research has shown us that women who do breast self-examination are not quite run of the mill. In the first place, they have a positive attitude to life and to BSE; they think it's a good thing to do, and they're right. They are likely to be better educated, younger, and belong to higher socioeconomic groups than women who don't examine their breasts. They also engage in other preventive health measures, such as cervical smears and dental checkups.

These women feel that breast cancer is the worst imaginable disease to affect women, but are optimistic about the likelihood of a cure with early treatment and believe it is something they can control by carrying out BSE regularly. They don't think that doing BSE will inevitably lead to finding a cancerous lump, and so they don't feel nervous about doing it. This is precisely the kind of approach and attitude you should try to cultivate.

WOMEN WHO DON'T

Unfortunately, nine out of ten women don't do BSE. There are many reasons for this. Good information on BSE is hard to find, and poor information tends to make women anxious. Even many health professionals who can tell you how to examine your breasts are unclear about what you're looking for because they themselves are uncertain. In addition, not every health educator is a good communicator, and you may end up with a confusing message. Many books and pamphlets tell you that you have to look for a change but don't explain what the precise changes are. You have no clear idea, therefore, of what you're searching for, which in itself provokes anxiety. Normal findings such as the premenstrual lumpiness of the breasts, for example, can be very frightening if you don't know that they are normal and can put you off BSE, because whatever is causing the lumps seems to be widespread.

It seems rather surprising in this day and age that women can actually be embarrassed about touching their own breasts, yet many women in their fifties and sixties, the age group for which breast cancer is most common, grew up with the view that it was somehow bad, except in the bath, for a woman to touch her own body. These women in particular may be astoundingly ignorant about their bodies.

I love examining my breasts – I'm proud of them, and I want them to be healthy. It makes me feel I'm in control of my life.
SUE, 25, MUSICIAN

A woman who considers that touching her breasts, let alone examining them, is somehow improper can remain unaware for a long time of dramatic changes in the breast, even large, ulcerating tumors.

Sometimes women are put off from performing BSE because they don't feel that there can be a positive outcome should they find something that needs medical attention. They therefore feel they are likely to be punished rather than rewarded for performing BSE. I don't want any woman reading this book to feel that if she's carrying out BSE regularly then she will inevitably turn up a worrying lump. This is not the case; in fact, we know it to be the opposite. Very few of the lumps that cause concern turn out to be cancerous. And even in the few cases where they do, most women with breast cancer don't die from it. Early detection of breast cancer vastly improves the chances of a cure. Rather than take a pessimistic point of view, I feel there's great room for optimism, because while you're doing BSE you're in control of your health.

WHEN TO DO BSE

Most experts advocating BSE suggest that you perform your examination at the same time every month – ideally in the week after your menstrual period – so that you have a consistent basis for comparison. When you're starting, however, I'm in favor of your examining your breasts at different times of the month because they will change in consistency and texture as you go through your monthly menstrual cycle (see below). I feel that all women should be aware of these changes and know how they feel to the touch. I also believe that it is better to perform BSE somewhat more frequently – say, every two weeks instead of once a month – in a low-key, relaxed way so that it quickly becomes a habit and part of normal life.

You should not feel tyrannized by BSE. However, becoming familiar with your breasts will help you provide appropriate care. If you find that the idea of breast examination makes you anxious, go along regularly to your doctor, say every three months, so that he or she can perform the examination for you and, if appropriate, take advantage of other early detection techniques such as mammograms (see p.64).

NORMAL LUMPINESS

Most women find that their breasts acquire what can only be described as lumpiness in the second half of the menstrual cycle, and this becomes easier to feel just prior to menstruation. Normal lumpiness is palpable throughout the breast tissue rather than concentrated in one spot. The lumps are very tiny and discrete – about the size, shape, and texture of an orange pit – and they may be tender if squeezed. This is because they are swollen milk glands, ready to develop into lactating glands should pregnancy occur.

If you examine your breasts again during the week after menstruation, you will find that these tiny lumps simply fade away as the glands shrink back. Once you've gotten used to these cyclical changes in your breasts, there's no need to examine them frequently; once or twice a month will suffice.

The first time I felt all those little lumps I almost flipped – then I thought if there are so many they can't be anything to be afraid of.

TRACEY, 35, PERSONNEL MANAGER

BREAST SELF-EXAMINATION

*There are two elements to breast self-examination:
looking and feeling (palpation). You will need a warm
place where you can have some privacy and be free from
interruptions. Just before going to bed is a good time,
or when you are about to have a bath or shower.*

LOOKING AT THE BREASTS

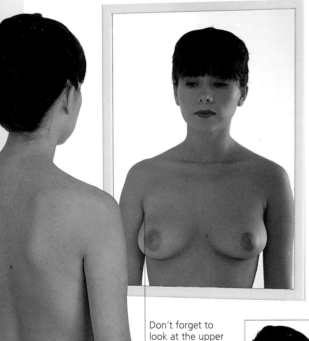

1 Undress to the waist and stand or sit in front of a mirror. Look at each breast carefully for changes in appearance, size, or the color of the nipples, a difference in level between the nipples, patches of eczema, or dimpling of the skin.

Don't forget to look at the upper part of the breast that leads into the armpit

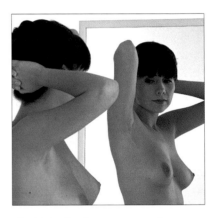

2 Raise both your arms above your head. Turn to one side so you can see your breasts in profile, and repeat your observations. Do the same for the other side.

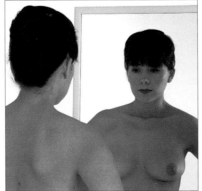

3 Place your hands firmly on your hips and press in hard. You should feel your chest muscles tense. Repeat your observations.

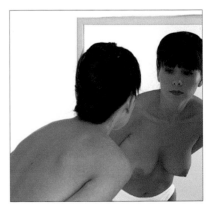

4 Now lean forward. Look again for dimpling or puckering of the skin, a change in outline of the breasts, or retraction of the nipple.

FEELING THE BREASTS

1 Lie back in a relaxed position and put your right arm behind your head. This shifts the breast tissue underneath your arm towards the center of your chest, giving you better access to it and making it easier for you to palpate. If you have very large breasts, you may need to put a pillow under your left shoulder.

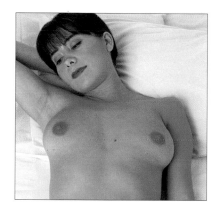

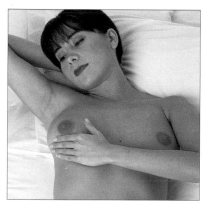

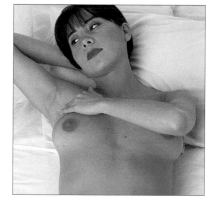

2 With a firm touch, examine your right breast with your left hand. You can use any of the patterns of palpation shown on the right or a pattern of your own, as long as it's systematic.

Use the sensitive pads of your fingertips, keeping your fingers parallel to the skin of the breast

3 Check your armpit and along the top of your collarbone for lumps (swollen lymph nodes).

4 Put your left hand behind your head and, using your right hand, examine your left breast in the same way. Remember to check the armpit and collarbone.

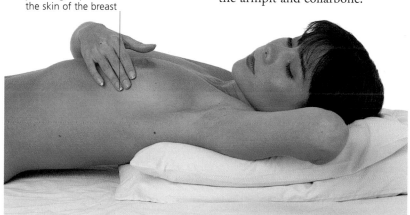

PATTERNS OF PALPATION

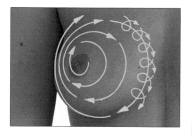

Concentric circles
Start with a large circle around the outside of the breast, making smaller circles with your fingers as you work your way around the breast. Work inward in rings until you reach the nipple.

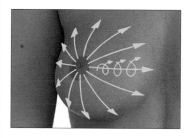

Radial pattern
Mentally divide the breast into a clock pattern. Work out from the nipple toward 12 o' clock, then 1, 2, 3 o' clock and so on, until you have checked the whole breast.

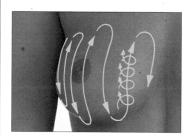

Up and down
Imagine the breast as a series of vertical bands, and work your way up and down each one. Move your fingers in small circles as you work around the breast.

YOUR FINDINGS

What you are looking for above all is a *change* in your breasts. You won't be able to recognize change, however, until you've examined your breasts a few times and established what is normal for you. Here are some of the things you may find in your breasts that are all quite normal and healthy:

Lumps and pseudolumps You may find all kinds of subtle changes within your breasts. I can almost guarantee that a subtle change is not a dangerous one. Cancer is not subtle, so don't panic over a lump that is extremely tiny and discrete, particularly if its size varies over your monthly cycle. Remember, your breasts may be lumpy naturally or premenstrually (see p.42).

Women who lose a lot of weight lose fat from the breasts as well, and this often makes the natural lumpiness more evident. The breastbone (between your breasts) makes joints at either edge with the ribs that may be prominent. If you're very thin, one of the hard lumps that you feel could simply be breast tissue felt over the end of a rib.

There may be a swelling of breast tissue between the nipple and the armpit or right above the nipple; there's more breast tissue here than in other areas of the breast (see p.37). Both of these areas are more likely to swell up and become tender in the premenstrual period. There is also a ridge of tissue in the lower part of the breast that feels thicker and more lumpy than other parts of the breast. Under the nipple you will be able to feel a hollow spot where the milk ducts rise to the surface.

If you've had any kind of infection in your breasts or any cause for surgical intervention, there will almost certainly be scar tissue that will always remain as a palpable lump or ridge. Even a biopsy will leave a scar. (If your doctor examines your breasts, remember to mention this and the date when it occurred, otherwise it may cause concern and the possibility of having to undergo further and unnecessary tests.)

Pain Soreness and discomfort are extremely common in women's breasts (see p.124). In the vast majority of cases they are connected with menstrual hormones and very rarely are symptoms of cancer. If soreness persists or if it is causing you problems, however, your doctor may be able to help. One promising treatment is to take evening primrose oil over a period of months.

SIGNIFICANT CHANGES

Once you have been practicing BSE long enough to get used to what is normal in your breasts, you will need to be on the alert for any changes that need a doctor's attention. There are several characteristic changes that might be of concern. First, here are some things you might observe while *looking* at your breasts:

Normal findings
When examining your breasts you may find changes that cause you concern. Many of these things, however, are quite normal and healthy and are shown below. If you are at all worried about any changes, consult your doctor at once.

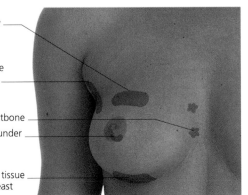

Pad of slightly thicker tissue

Bulge of tissue in axillary tail

Knobs where ribs join with edge of breastbone

Hollow spot under the nipple

Ridge of firm tissue under the breast

- change in the size of either breast

- change in the color or texture of the skin

- new dimpling or puckering of the skin over the breast and nipple, or change in the breast outline

- change in the appearance of the nipple, such as redness, scaling, crusting, or drawing in

- discharge or bleeding from the nipple

When *palpating,* you are really looking for only one thing: a new, discrete lump that is constant in size and doesn't vary with your menstrual cycle. The lump may be attached to the skin, causing it to pucker, or it may be fixed to the tissues deeper in the breast. If you feel such a lump, your next step should be to examine the armpit to see whether or not any of your lymph nodes are swollen and then to run your finger along the top of your collarbone to see if there are swollen nodes in that area as well. There are three main criteria for deciding that a lump needs medical investigation – please bear in mind that this is not the same thing as saying that the lump must necessarily be cancerous.

- The lump is new.

- It is very distinct, not just a thickening of the breast tissue.

- It remains unchanged throughout one or two menstrual cycles.

If you find something but can't decide whether it's serious or not, see your doctor anyway, if only to set your mind at rest. The vast majority of lumps detected by BSE are not cancerous and are quite normal.

WHAT TO DO IF YOU FIND A LUMP

First check the same part of the other breast. If what you have found is symmetrical, it's just the way your breasts are made; and nothing for you to worry about. If the lump is asymmetrical, don't panic. Phone your doctor to make an appointment for a breast examination at the earliest opportunity. If he or she is at all worried, you will be referred very quickly to a specialist, and further tests will be done (see p.159). Make a mental note of exactly where the lump is located in your breast, and try not to keep re-examining the lump to see if it's still there or if it's tender.

Now sit down, phone your best friend, and ask her to come around right away. However rational you think you can be about it, you will be glad of moral support before, during, and after your medical appointment. Keep on reminding yourself that the majority of breast lumps are not cancerous.

DISCHARGE

Some leaflets and books about BSE tell you to squeeze your nipples and check for discharge. You should not do this as part of your breast examination routine. Squeezing the nipple can create discharge where there was none before, because it increases the hormone prolactin (see p.92) in the body, which in turn causes the breasts to produce liquid (though not full milk).

The way to check for discharge is simply to examine your clothes and you should do this at least every time you do BSE. Discharge is only a cause for concern if it appears without any squeezing of the nipples, if it is persistent, or if it's from one nipple only (squeeze your other nipple to check this); then you should consult your doctor (see p.133).

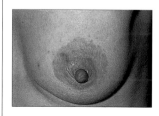

Eczema
Redness or scaling on the areola may be eczema, particularly if you have it elsewhere. You should always consult your doctor.

SCREENING

While breast self-examination is recommended for all women at all stages of their lives, additional checks are advisable for older women, whose risk of breast cancer is higher, and for women in other high-risk groups – with breast cancer in the family, for instance. Screening programs are offered from time to time in various communities, often at relatively low cost. Screening involves a physical breast examination – a doctor will examine your breasts in the same way that you do at home for BSE (see p.58) – and a mammogram (see below), which can pick up smaller abnormalities than a physical examination.

Many women are apprehensive about going to these clinics, just as they are about BSE – when what they really fear, of course, is that the examination may reveal a breast lump. Of course you can decide that you don't wish to be screened for the early detection of breast cancer; you must make up your own mind whether regular screening will cause you undue anxiety.

In deciding, remember there is now clear evidence that early detection by screening and treatment cuts down the number of women dying from breast cancer. Studies performed in Sweden and the U.S. have shown that screening can reduce by up to a third deaths from breast cancer in women between the ages of 50 and 65. Early detection automatically means earlier treatment and so increases the chances of a full recovery if a lump is found that turns out to be breast cancer. Early detection also means you can have greater choice in how your cancer will be treated.

It's understandable to be anxious about having regular mammograms but it's reassuring to know that most mammograms are clear, showing no evidence of cancer. Only a minority show suspicious changes, and most of these turn out to be quite harmless when examined further. If you are referred by your doctor for a hospital test after screening, try if possible to think positively and remind yourself that you will probably be one of the 99 women out of every 100 screened who are found not to have cancer.

MAMMOGRAPHY

A mammogram is an X-ray of the breast, though the X-rays used are rather different from those that examine the internal organs; they are low-dose and designed to show up the soft tissue of the breasts very well. A mammogram is so refined that it can pick up small cancers and other abnormalities that neither you nor your doctor can feel on manual examination. Given all the benefits of screening, it is hard to believe that there could be any criticism of mammography, but four have been suggested:

• A negative result could create a false sense of security and could discourage women from examining their own breasts; women need to be made aware of the benefits of self-examination.

• A very few mammograms may miss cancers and give false negative results. Self-examination or examination by a doctor may pick up problems.

I felt ambivalent really. You know, glad that nothing was found but also scared that next time I have a mammogram something will show up.

CLAIRE, 53,
TOUR OPERATOR

MAMMOGRAPHIC SCREENING

To have a mammogram done, you'll be asked to strip to the waist and to remove any deodorant or talc from your breasts. The reason for this is that they may show up as microcalcifications (see p.66). You will then be asked to stand in front of the machine, and the radiologist will compress your breast between two plates. The procedure is described as painless but it is not without a degree of discomfort, particularly if the plates are cold; the sensation lasts no more than 10 or 15 seconds, however, so it's easily bearable. Two views of each breast will usually be taken.

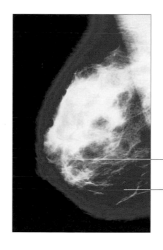

MAMMOGRAM
In this normal breast, glandular tissue shows up in yellow, while the fatty part of the breast is in red. The lower proportion of breast tissue is typical of a mature woman's breasts.

— Dense glandular tissue

— Fatty tissue

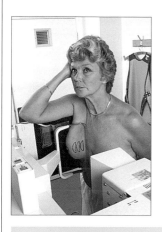

OBTAINING THE IMAGE
Each breast in turn will be compressed between two plates (left) so as to get a good image.

INTERPRETATION
A radiologist (right) experienced in interpreting mammograms scrutinizes each image for any sign of abnormality.

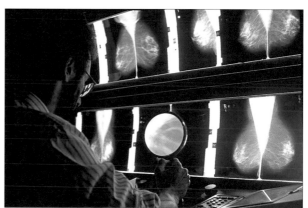

• A mammogram will sometimes pick out as suspicious an abnormality that in fact is not cancer at all; a false positive is estimated to occur in about 1 in every 100 mammograms. Getting a second opinion and having further tests should resolve uncertainties.

• Some people worry that the radiation from a mammogram may cause breast cancer, but the doses of X-rays are minute, so the risk is only very slight.

A final thought is that screening turns otherwise well women into patients undergoing medical tests, making them aware of the possibility of ill health and also of being labeled as diseased, something we would all like to avoid.

WHO IS IT FOR?

Mammograms are not performed with the same frequency in all age groups. Breast cancer is comparatively rare in women under the age of 40, and so it is only after 40 that annual mammograms are recommended. Women who are in high-risk groups will be encouraged to have annual or biannual mammograms at an earlier age than usual (see p.64). In England, mammography is offered to women over 50 every three years, though there is currently some debate about this, and the frequency may be increased to every two years. The age to begin getting mammograms and at what frequency are currently under debate. The American Cancer Society recommends annual mammograms after age 40. Since the risks and benefits of mammography are affected by many variables, you will probably want to discuss your decision with your doctor.

Mammography is less effective in women under 50, because their breast tissue is more dense, and abnormalities don't show up so well. It is still more sensitive than BSE, however, which is why it can be used as a diagnostic tool: to investigate a lump found in physical examination, for example, or to look for further lumps when one has already been found.

Mammography is most reliable for the examination of large breasts because they allow a greater degree of contrast for clear and more accurate X-ray pictures. A trained radiologist is able to pick out even small cysts and tiny tumors, however, whatever the size of your breasts.

THE RESULTS

The films will be developed and examined by a radiologist specializing in the interpretation of mammograms. You may receive the results at the time of mammography or in a few days. Most women will be told that they're fine and just need regular screening; a small number will be asked to come back for further tests. This can be worrisome, but the chances of getting the all-clear are still high. Although mammograms are worthwhile for detecting small lumps, they're not very useful for determining what the precise characteristics of a lump are, so extra tests may be needed.

Your first mammogram will act as a baseline against which all subsequent mammograms will be compared. It is very helpful for your doctor and most reassuring for you to see the same result time after time, and it is also useful for you to become familiar with the inconsistencies and idiosyncracies of your breasts. In my own case, I have a particularly dense shadow in one of my breasts, but it has never changed over fifteen years, and although it caused concern the first time it showed up on mammogram, since then it has just been noted and checked each time the screening is performed.

Microcalcifications These are tiny deposits of calcium that show up as very fine specks on a mammogram. They may be quite normal, and many women have them, but because they have been linked with cancer in a small number of cases, the radiologist will always mention if they are present. They are only worrisome if they suddenly appear in a cluster in one breast. If it's your first mammogram, then of course your doctor can't tell if they're new and so may recommend a further mammogram in about six months' time, which is long enough to see if there is any change. If the pattern of microcalcification is very abnormal, a biopsy (see p.160) will be carried out at once.

Lumps If your mammogram shows any kind of lump, then further tests will be necessary. A lump that's large enough to feel easily with your fingers can be aspirated – that is, a fine needle inserted and some of the tissue drawn off (this is called fine-needle aspiration cytology, or FNAC – see p.127).

If the lump is fluid-filled, then it's a cyst (see p.131) and perfectly harmless; your doctor will draw off the fluid with the needle and send off a specimen for laboratory tests. If it's solid, some of the cells that have been drawn off will be smeared on a glass slide, stained, and examined in the lab.

If the lump isn't easy to feel, you will probably have an ultrasound scan (see below) to determine whether it's a solid lump or a cyst. Either way it may be investigated with fine-needle aspiration cytology, as described above, or cutting-needle biopsy with a slightly larger needle (see p.160). When a lump can't be felt, both these specimens are taken under stereotactic guidance on an ultrasound screen, so that the tumor can be precisely located.

REASONS WOMEN GIVE FOR NOT GETTING MAMMOGRAMS

"I examine my breasts fairly regularly and I've never found anything to worry about. Besides, my doctor's never mentioned it."

The point of mammograms is to find lumps before they become large enough to be discoverable by BSE; mammography can detect abnormalities that are too small to be felt by you or your doctor. You should get screened whether or not you have any breast symptoms. Don't leave it to your doctor to recommend; ask about it.

"What about all that radiation going into your breast?"

The technology used in mammograms has improved since they were introduced, and the most up-to-date machinery uses a very low dose of radiation – comparable to a routine dental X-ray. Given the infrequency of screening mammograms, the tiny amounts of radiation involved, and the ability of mammograms to detect very small abnormalities, the benefits far outweigh any risk of radiation.

"I've just never gotten around to it."

Because mammograms can detect lumps too small to feel – as small as ¼ inch (0.5 centimeters) – they give us a great advantage in fighting cancer. Early detection vastly improves the outlook for women who do get breast cancer, so it's important to get mammograms regularly, especially if you're over 50.

"I know I should go, but the thought that they might find something terrifies me."

Of 1,000 women who receive a mammogram, 990 will be given the all-clear. Of the remaining ten, nine will be found to have only benign lumps. Most important, the one woman in every 1,000 who is found to have a malignant lump will have greatly improved her outlook by taking action so that the disease is detected early. By getting screened you are not inviting disaster; you are giving yourself the best chance of health.

"It hurts, doesn't it?"

Mammography is uncomfortable, but very few women (about 6 percent, according to one study) actually find it painful. Your breasts are compressed for only about 15 seconds, so the discomfort doesn't last very long. If you are prone to premenstrual breast tenderness, it's a good idea to arrange your screening session for the week after menstruation to minimize the possibility of pain.

"I'm too embarrassed to have my breasts examined by a stranger – it all sounds so undignified."

Given the proven life-saving benefits of mammography, it is important that you overcome your inhibitions and consult a doctor as soon as possible. You should remember that you are only one of thousands of women whose bodies the screening team sees every year. You have nothing to feel embarrassed about, and you can expect to be treated in a sensitive and professional manner. Ask to see a female doctor if you prefer.

OTHER IMAGING TECHNIQUES

Mammography is the most widely used method of imaging the breast, but there are some other techniques that you may come across, particularly if you are referred for further tests after a screening mammogram.

XERO-MAMMOGRAPHY

Xero-mammography requires different equipment from the standard X-ray machine that takes a mammogram. It is not necessarily any more accurate than mammography; it just gives a different end-product – an image on paper rather than on film. Accuracy of interpretation depends on the experience of the radiologist, whatever method is used.

ULTRASOUND

Many of us have come across ultrasonic scans during pregnancy, where they are used to check on the health of the developing baby. Ultrasound can produce a picture very similar to an X-ray photograph. The patterns are produced by the echoes of sound waves, which vary in intensity according to the solidity of the tissue that they bounce off. Ultrasound can be particularly useful when examining very dense breasts, so it's good for younger women and can detect very small lumps that can't yet be felt, particularly tiny cysts. It's very accurate with larger, palpable lumps, and it can distinguish between fluid-filled and solid lumps.

Ultrasound is very accurate at pinpointing ill-defined tumors that have shown up on mammogram but can't be felt. Indeed, it is used to locate a tumor stereotactically prior to surgery (see p.175). It's also useful to monitor the progress of noncancerous lumps without the X-ray load of repeated mammograms. Finally, it detects calcification (see p.66) and can reveal the blood supply to a tumor – a rich supply is characteristic of cancerous lumps.

Ultrasound is painless. The skin of the breast is lubricated, and a small instrument that emits sound waves is run over it. We know from extensive research involving pregnant women that there are no harmful side effects.

THERMOGRAPHY

Less familiar than X-rays or ultrasound, thermography is never a first-line investigation, as other procedures yield much more information; it's usually used as a supportive investigation to manual examination and mammography.

Rapidly growing and dividing tissue such as cancer has a higher temperature than the tissue surrounding it. Thermography works by mapping out the temperatures in different tissues, so a growing cyst or a tumor will show up on a thermogram as a more intense area of heat than its surroundings. To have a thermogram done, the patient undresses and holds her arms up or stretched out from the body to allow the breast skin to cool. Photographs are then taken of the breasts from different angles with an infrared camera. Thermography isn't as accurate as mammography because some cancers don't give off heat, while others may be too deep in the breast to show up.

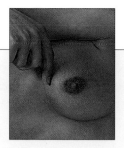

CHAPTER FOUR

THE
SEXUAL
BREAST

Throughout history the female breast
has been a potent symbol of sexuality. Its
role in sexual arousal is a dual one, since
it is both exciting to men and a source of
erotic pleasure for women. Despite
changing fashions, the public and private
image of the breast remains one of
sensuality, femininity, and fertility.

THE PROVOCATIVE BREAST

We live in a world where the breast is a potent sex symbol. Most female breasts, whether clothed or not, are clearly visible and serve as a focus not only for sexual arousal but sexual titillation. It's natural for a woman who feels attracted to a man, and wishes to interest and excite him, to display her breasts or use them as a weapon of sexual provocation. It's natural, too, for a man to be attracted to and excited by a woman's breasts.

DRESSING THE BREAST

Today's breast-conscious woman is only one in a long line of women who, throughout the ages, have treated the breast as a sexual provocateur. Minoan women in Bronze Age Crete bared their breasts, the women of ancient Egypt covered them with gossamer-fine cotton, and Greek women adorned themselves with see-through linen. In many respects, our generation is restrained compared with the women we see in eighteenth-century French paintings; their breasts were blatantly uplifted by empire-line dresses and barely covered by the flimsiest wisp of silk.

Anyone brave enough can go the whole way and wear a completely transparent top with a bra clearly visible underneath: the quintessence of the provocative breast is no longer nakedness, as it was in the topless and braless years. It's not surprising, therefore, that bras and corsets are being assertively worn as overgarments and form the basis of many 1990s dress designs. What goes under the dress is as important, at least in the bedroom, as what goes over it. Not only are there bra styles to divide, uplift, maximize, and push up (see p.56), but they are fashioned in the most delicious fabrics and colors, from the gently feminine to the aggressively audacious, to suit a woman's every mood. In addition, newspaper advertisements testify to bras in rubber and shiny materials to tease fetishists, catering to all tastes.

Greek women
The women of ancient Greece frequently wore transparent linen to enhance the allure of their breasts.

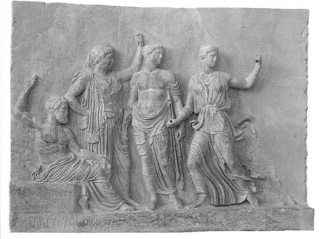

CHANGING FASHIONS

The fashionable breast most typical of the 1980s was perhaps the aggressive breast – sharp, pointed, and clothed in material resembling steel. No softness and nurturing here; the breasts were more like weapons. Such breasts sent out messages of "hands off," "keep back," "don't meddle with me" – signals that mean "I'm just fine by myself, no man needed," the badge of the ultimate independent, feminist woman. This look was typified by the conical bra worn by Madonna in the late 1980s.

In the 1990s the breast is softer, but still highly visible: at the start of the decade, the fashion industry announced that breasts were "back in fashion," and a comparison between recent fashion magazines and those of ten years ago will show the difference. The "ideal figure" being sold to women in the 1990s is still well toned and athletic, but with more generous curves and a definite cleavage. This combination of a slim, athletic body with large breasts is physically implausible – as one model put it, "Nature doesn't make women like that." Even so, the phenomenal renaissance of the push-up bra testifies to women's efforts to conform to this new ideal.

It is curious, but nonetheless true, that there should be fashions in breast types. What remains constant, however, is women's use of the breasts as part of the armory of sex appeal.

BREAST ORNAMENTATION

Whenever society encourages or at least allows the breasts to be displayed, the opportunity exists to adorn them. In Europe in the latter half of the sixteenth century, women's exposed breasts were as heavily made up as their faces, and with the same pernicious substance – ceruse, a poisonous lead compound that made the skin look radiantly white. Eventually, however, it corroded the skin and was absorbed into the bloodstream. At this time, too, middle-aged women would paint a tracery of blue veins on their breasts in imitation of the fragile, transparent skin of much younger women.

During sexual excitement, women's nipples become suffused with blood, swell, and become deeper in color, like their lips. Thus, just as red lipstick is a sexual signal to men because it simulates this, in the same way the nipples and areola can be rouged and displayed under filmy garments. It's possible to keep a nipple erect by painting it with nail polish. This is a trick used by fashion models and striptease dancers, but not recommended for general use.

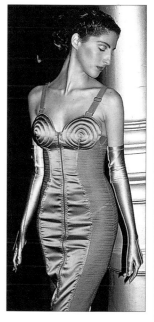

Aggressive breast
This designer outfit depicts the aggressive breast that became fashionable during the 1980s.

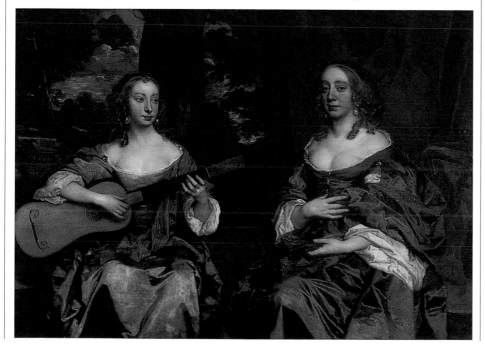

Prominent breast
During the seventeenth century breasts were highly provocative, with women wearing uplifting bodices and plunging necklines.

THE SENSUAL BREAST

The breast is a secondary sexual characteristic in more ways than one. The first and obvious one is in an anatomical sense, because the presence of breasts is the visual badge of our gender difference from men.

In a quite separate and physiological sense, the breast is a secondary sexual characteristic as an erogenous zone, greatly sensitive to sexual arousal and undergoing many changes during sexual excitement and the achievement of orgasm (see p.78). The effects of arousal can be clearly seen as deepening in the color of the skin over the breast, areola, and nipple, and felt in the form of substantial swelling and turgidity of the breast and nipple.

A DIGRESSION ON EVOLUTION

Human female breasts are uniquely large among mammals. In the first place, they are a permanent feature in human adult females, whereas in other mammals they appear only when there are infants to be fed. In the second, and as an inevitable consequence of the first, it is only in humans that the breasts feature in sexual activity at all. In considering the sexual and sensual properties of the breast it is natural to ask why this is so and how it came about.

We do not know at what stage in human evolution the enlarged female breast developed because, as it consists entirely of soft tissue, it leaves no fossil remains. We can learn something, however, by looking at the most ancient of all representations of the human form – "Venus" or "mother goddess" figurines. Although their sexual characteristics, including the breasts, are grossly exaggerated, it is nonetheless clear that the human female breast was established in recognizable form well over a thousand generations ago.

Hidden ovulation Charles Darwin's theory of natural selection states that we develop, maintain, and pass on to our offspring those characteristics that best enable us to adapt to our environments. Since a feature that is selected has to benefit those who have it, we must ask ourselves what benefit an enlarged breast confers. An interesting area of speculation centers around the hidden ovulation of the human female.

Sexual reproduction demands that a live sperm fertilize a live ovum, and since most females do not ovulate continually, it is vital that the sexual act coincide with ovulation. Species have developed varied and wonderful ways of ensuring this, and for the most part they depend for their success on the female advertising the fact not only of her fertility but of her receptivity. This in turn motivates the males to impregnate her. The signals used take many forms, but in mammals they appeal predominantly to sight, smell, or both. The human female, however, does not show any outward sign of being "in heat." If we were asked to tell which three of any dozen women were ovulating, we would not know how to go about it. In this regard, human females are different not only from other mammals but also from virtually every other species that relies on sexual reproduction.

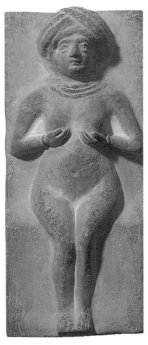

Earth goddess
This Sumerian earth goddess from 2,000 BC emphasises the rounded forms of the female breasts and hips.

So how do humans ensure that they mate at the correct moment? What signals does the female give to the male to indicate her fertile state? The answer, of course, is that she does not give any. How can she? She herself does not know. She does not even know in the way that animals "know" – that is, in being compelled by instinct to act in certain ways. In humans, therefore, sexual intercourse has to occur sufficiently frequently so that, if only by chance, sperm will meet the ovum at the optimum time.

Human sexual arousal Where there is no signal to stimulate arousal, the male must either be in a permanent state of semi-arousal or be capable of being easily aroused. Mating is more likely to succeed, too, if the female is eager, otherwise penetration will be difficult. Sexual arousal in a woman triggers the production of vaginal secretions that facilitate penetration. As another inducement to frequent sexual intercourse, women are capable of achieving an orgasm; no other female of any species is thought to have this capacity.

Can we infer a connection, then, between the opulent human breast, which we know is not related to milk production, and the hidden nature of human ovulation? If the easily aroused male needs only the most unsophisticated signal of sexual availability, did the breast come to be seen as such a signal during the course of human evolution? Given that the female has her own sexual agenda, is the breast one of the mechanisms through which she secures the arousal of the relevant male? It seems a reasonable hypothesis that the human breast is the result of sexual selection – the passing on of any trait or characteristic that helps to increase an individual's chance of mating. If we accept this, it follows that the potency of the breast as a sex symbol is not just cultural but fundamental to human sexuality.

BREAST SENSITIVITY

The breasts make an especially powerful contribution to sexual excitement, being endowed as they are with two separate sets of nerves. The first set, the sensory nerves, are purely tactile, and when stimulated lead to arousal and a general heightening of sexual excitement. The second set, however, are connected to the deeper autonomic nervous system, which supplies most of the internal organs. The autonomic nerves are responsible for a range of unconscious or involuntary body functions. Through connections in the solar plexus, the autonomic nerves (see p.39) send signals to the clitoris and can bring about clitoral excitement and erection, even though the clitoris itself remains untouched and unstimulated. Some women find that these nervous connections are so highly developed that stimulation of the breasts and nipples can bring about clitoral orgasm.

THE BREAST AS AN EROGENOUS ZONE

Certain areas of the body, especially parts of the skin, are particularly sensitive sexually. These are called erogenous zones. Although both men and women have erogenous zones, women have more, and they are more important to the

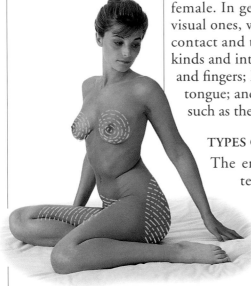

Most sensitive areas
Erogenous zones vary, but for most women the genitals, breasts, buttocks, and inner thighs are very responsive to touch, strokes, and kisses.

female. In general, men are aroused by psychological stimuli, particularly visual ones, whereas women are usually strongly aroused only with physical contact and touch stimuli. Erogenous zones may be stimulated by various kinds and intensities of touch: caresses or even light slapping with the hands and fingers; licking, kissing, nibbling, and sucking with the mouth, lips, and tongue; and rubbing with parts of the body that are themselves erogenous, such as the penis or the breasts.

TYPES OF EROGENOUS ZONE

The erogenous zones can be classified as primary, secondary, and tertiary. The most important of the primaries are the external genital organs for women. Other primary erogenous zones include the lips, buttocks, and breasts, especially the nipples. Secondary zones are those with sexual connotations derived from society or that are specific to the relationship between two people. Such zones could include the ears, eyelids, upper legs – particularly the inner thighs – and any part of the skin that is normally covered. Among individual couples, secondary erogenous zones can vary widely. Tertiary erogenous zones are those parts of the body that on occasion feel sexy when touched, for example the arms and hands.

The region of the clitoris is a woman's most sensitive zone. This is followed by her mouth, which when stimulated can set her whole body alight and, as with the breasts and nipples, can even have a direct effect in arousing her clitoris and vagina. A woman's face has several erogenous zones too, including her hairline, forehead, temples, eyebrows, eyelids, and cheeks.

WHAT MAKES THE BREAST EROGENOUS?

The main reason that certain areas of the skin are known as erogenous zones is because they are very sensitive. Their sensitivity is due to a rich supply of sensory nerve endings, particularly those that pick up touch. (Others detect pleasure, pain, and temperature.) The richest supplies of sensory nerve endings are in the lips and the skin surrounding the mouth, the fingertips, the areola and the nipple, and all the external genital organs. In a sexual situation, the touch stimuli become sexual stimuli.

An important though secondary factor affecting the conversion of touch stimuli to sexual stimuli is the emotional involvement of the woman and the intensity of the situation. If the emotional component is very high, touch of almost any part of the body becomes sexually stimulating.

The breasts' natural qualifications as primary erogenous zones are further boosted by the eroticization of the breast that is so deeply rooted in our culture and may even be fundamental to human nature. Given the profoundly pleasurable sensations that most women experience when their breasts are stimulated, and the importance attached by most men to the breasts in their assessment of sexual attractiveness, it is not surprising that women regard their breasts as vital to and a visible sign of their sexuality and femininity.

GETTING IN TOUCH WITH YOUR BREASTS

Given that the breast is unquestionably a sex organ capable of arousal, it's a pity to miss out on the pleasure that it can bring. The majority of women caress themselves while masturbating, but if you haven't and are unaware of how pleasurable manipulation of the breasts can be, it's never too late to try.

Using fantasy may help; it can be extremely valuable for rehearsing or experimenting with unfamiliar experiences. By using your imagination, for example, you can explore new sexual techniques before you actually put them into practice. You can experiment without fear of embarrassment and have a trial run before you ask your partner to cooperate.

The first step is to prepare as though for deep relaxation, which means finding a warm, quiet, and comfortable place to lie, dressed in something soft and loose. (You may want to take a warm bath first.) With the lights dimmed, lie down, close your eyes, and imagine as pleasant a scene as you can in a favorite location. Next concentrate on your breathing: breathe in as deeply as you can to a count of five, hold your breath for two or three seconds, then exhale very slowly. While you're breathing, think of nothing but what you're doing; concentrate on the air entering and expanding your lungs and then leaving them as they deflate. This should slow down your breathing rate by about half, which will engender a great feeling of relaxation and tranquillity.

Now imagine your body to be filling up with warm honey. Visualize the honey flowing into various parts of your body, starting with your head and neck and spreading down over your shoulders and into your arms. Imagine that the honey is flowing into your breasts and nipples, making them swollen and tense. Take your mind over a guided tour of your breasts, feeling every part intimately. Watch yourself in the mirror if you like. Think very hard about what you're experiencing, and concentrate on the pleasure.

EXPLORING YOUR BREASTS

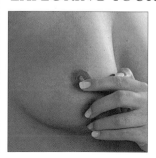

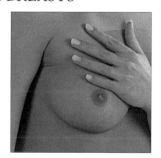

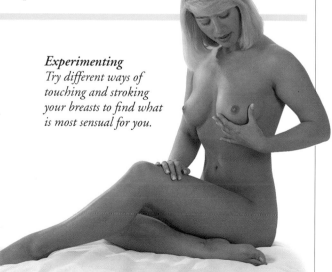

Experimenting
Try different ways of touching and stroking your breasts to find what is most sensual for you.

Pressing
Nipples and areolae can be stimulated by gently scratching them or pressing them with your fingertips.

Caressing
Gently squeeze and fondle your breasts with the palm of your hand.

THE BREASTS AND MASTURBATION

For most girls, masturbation is an introduction to sex and the means to their first orgasms. It helps them to know how they function sexually and to form preferences, and may contribute to successful sexual intercourse. Two-thirds of girls masturbate by the time they're 16. An adolescent girl engaging in masturbation will notice the swelling of her breasts and the erection of her nipples and may absentmindedly or knowingly caress them herself. For most women, breast stimulation greatly heightens sexual excitement and may be enough to bring about or at least contribute to an orgasm. Many women love the sight and feel of their own breasts in a nonsexual way in any case, and caressing them can be simply consoling and comforting – part of how a woman can enjoy her body. Here are some women's accounts of how their breasts play a part in arousal when they masturbate:

"I masturbate lying in bed at night. First I take my nightclothes off and just relax. I like to touch my breasts softly and stimulate them."

"I moisten my fingertips with my tongue and lightly touch my breasts so it feels as if a tongue were licking them."

"I have had an orgasm while playing with my breasts on several occasions."

"I stroke my clitoris until I begin to feel excited, then I use my other hand to stimulate my nipples at the same time. I have hardly ever reached orgasm without simultaneous nipple stimulation."

THE BREASTS AND FOREPLAY

Sex is an escalating activity, starting off with touching and caressing and going on to kissing and foreplay. Foreplay is often much more important to women than to men. Men tend to become sexually aroused by thoughts, sights, and talking. Women are generally much less easily aroused by these things; in fact, they have a much narrower range of erotic stimuli than men. The majority of women need physical stimulation of the breasts, clitoris, and vagina to get them sexually aroused. What is more, this stimulation has to be continuous for sexual excitement to build.

It's true that women are more easily distracted during sexual foreplay than men. This is why women may find that they are listening for sounds or even going over tomorrow morning's shopping list if foreplay is not successful. A woman is most sexy when she feels most and thinks least.

For most women, sexual play involving the breasts is an enjoyable part of foreplay because the breasts are highly erotic and play a vital part in sexual excitement. Sucking, nibbling, licking, stroking, or gentle squeezing will all cause the nipples to become erect, a sign that a more sensitive phase of sexual excitement has been reached. Women do differ greatly, however, in their reactions to breast stimulation. Some women like their breasts, and the nipples in particular, to be pressed and bitten to the point of hurting, while others complain that men are too rough with their breasts during foreplay.

SEX PLAY

The vast majority of women are aroused by touch and will enjoy having their breasts caressed and stimulated in a variety of ways during foreplay and intercourse – indeed, for some women, breast stimulation is essential in helping them to reach orgasm.

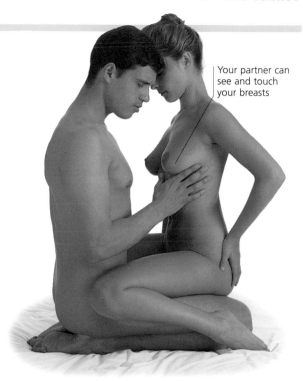

Your partner can see and touch your breasts

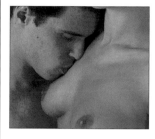

USING THE LIPS
Kissing, nibbling, and sucking are all good ways of stimulating the nipples.

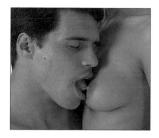

USING THE TONGUE
The warm, wet feel of her partner's tongue on a woman's breasts, and in particular the nipples, can be very arousing.

FRONT TO FRONT
If the man kneels and pulls his partner onto his thighs he can easily reach forward to stimulate her breasts.

FRONT TO BACK
The "spoons" position is one of the most comfortable. The man can reach round to stimulate the woman's breasts and clitoris.

Your partner can caress your breasts

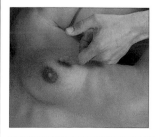

SCRATCHING
A man can experiment with the sensations his partner feels by gently drawing his fingernails across her breasts.

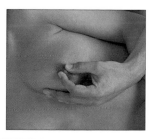

SQUEEZING
Some women enjoy more vigorous stimulation as well as gentle caresses.

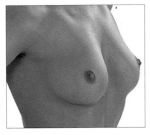

Erect nipple
One of the first signs of
sexual arousal in the
breasts is erection of the
nipples. Even inverted
nipples respond a little.

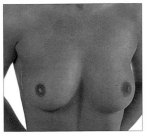

Sexual flush
During heightened sexual
arousal, blood vessels
dilate and the increased
flow of blood often results
in a pink rash, notably
across the chest.

SEXUAL RESPONSES

In 1931 sexual physiologists Theodore Van de Velde and Robert Dickinson first described changes in the breasts during sexual arousal and climax. Their description was simple, noting that the breast swelled with sexual excitement.

In the 1950s, William H. Masters and Virginia E. Johnson, as part of their in-depth study of sexual responses, described four phases of sexual response: excitement, the plateau phase, orgasm, and resolution. Among the many changes taking place in the body, they identified clear changes in the breast.

Excitement Erection of the nipple is the first sign in the breasts of increasing sexual excitement. Such erection occurs because the small muscle fibers that are within the nipple itself contract (see p.38). Both nipples rarely become erect at the same rate; one is usually ahead of the other in terms of turgidity and size. They can increase by as much as a centimeter in length and by half a centimeter in diameter. The larger the nipple in its resting state, the less it will increase in size when aroused.

One of the most marked changes in the breast as sexual excitement increases is the growth in volume as the blood vessels within it fill up; this is exactly similar to the mechanism that results in erection of the penis and is known as engorgement. This doesn't just occur underneath the surface; some of the dilated veins are visible on the skin. In the late part of the excitement phase the areola too becomes engorged, turning a deep rosy red color and becoming so swollen around the nipple that it may appear bruised.

Plateau phase As its name suggests, the plateau phase is a stage where sexual excitement, having initially increased, levels off before proceeding to orgasm. This may last much longer for men than for women – because women usually take longer than men to reach full arousal, the man remains at the plateau stage until the woman catches up and both partners are ready for penetration.

When a woman reaches the plateau phase, a pink mottling known as the sexual flush appears on her chest and sides and eventually the under-surface of the breasts. About three-quarters of all women show this flush on occasion, and as sexual tension mounts toward the end of the plateau phase, this measles-like rash can spread over the lower abdomen, shoulders, front and sides of the thighs, buttocks, and back. The color deepens and the spread widens just prior to the end of the plateau phase with orgasm. Here are some women's descriptions of how they feel at this stage:

"I feel an exquisite tension and a yearning in my breasts to be touched."

"I feel a heightened sensitivity all over and ache to be touched on my breasts, stomach, buttocks, and vagina."

"I am aware of every bit of my body, but especially my genitals, breasts, neck, stomach, mouth, and ears."

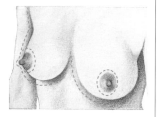

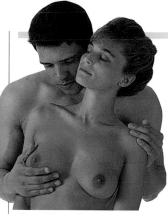

BREAST STIMULATION

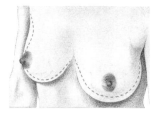

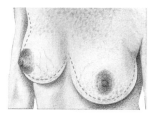

Fondling the breasts brings about several distinct stages of arousal.

EXCITEMENT
The nipples are erect, the breasts engorged, and the areolae are so swollen that they can look bruised.

PLATEAU
Just before orgasm, sexual arousal levels out and a pink rash (sexual flush) appears on the chest.

RESOLUTION
After orgasm, the sexual flush soon disappears and the breasts and areolae revert to their normal size.

Before sexual excitement resolves in orgasm, a breast that has never produced milk will increase in size by about a fifth to a quarter, while one that has does not usually show as clear an increase. This is because suckling promotes the drainage of blood from the breast, and engorgement cannot therefore take place. The more babies suckled, the less change there will be.

Orgasm There is no particular change in the breasts at the time of orgasm. The nipples stand erect, the areolae are swollen, and veins stand out boldly on the skin of the breasts, with the nonsuckled breast significantly bigger than in its unstimulated state and the sexual flush widely distributed and deep pink.

Resolution The sexual flush disappears rapidly with orgasm, fading from body parts in reverse order of its appearance. The swelling of the areolae subsides quickly so that the nipples appear to regain their full erection and are said to be in a state of post-orgasmic erection. This, however, is only an impression created because the areolae and breasts quickly shrink to their normal size, leaving the erect nipple proud and stiff for a few minutes longer. This is particularly clear in a woman who has never breastfed, but less so in a woman who has suckled. Nonsuckled breasts may take five to ten minutes after orgasm to return to their unexcited state, and the nipples even longer.

RESPONSES IN THE MALE BREAST

Sexual excitement in men does not cause any consistent response in the male breast. Nipple erection quite frequently occurs in the late excitement phase, however, and lasts through the remainder of the sexual cycle. In 60 percent of men studied by Masters and Johnson, further swelling of the nipple followed in the plateau phase. Once nipple swelling is established, it may take more than an hour after ejaculation to subside. Nipple erection can develop even if the nipple is not directly touched.

PREGNANCY

Breast arousal is the same in a pregnant woman as in a nonpregnant woman, and given that the breasts are already swollen and tender, this can result in quite severe pain and tenderness. Changes in size during sexual excitement are usually confined to the first half of pregnancy, however. By the last trimester, breast volume has increased by roughly a third, and even high states of sexual excitement don't provoke any further increase in breast size.

LACTATION

Breasts that are swollen with milk do not increase in size at all during sexual excitement, but some women may respond to sexual stimulation by losing milk in uncontrolled spurts. Milk will run from both nipples simultaneously during and immediately after orgasm, whether it occurs during sexual intercourse or masturbation. The majority of men are not put off by this, and some men find lactating breasts a real turn-on. Many men will also want to taste their partners' milk and enjoy doing so.

THE BREASTS AND LABOR

Nipple stimulation has been found to be effective in helping a pregnant woman go into labor when her baby is overdue. Stimulation, which can be done manually, orally, or with a breast pump, causes the release of the hormone oxytocin, which in turn causes the uterus to contract. This is the same as the mechanism whereby oxytocin helps the uterus return to its normal size after birth. The nipples should not be stimulated for more than a few minutes, however, as prolonged stimulation has been associated with fetal distress. First used in the 1830s, this method is now adopted by women interested in a drug-free labor.

THE OLDER BREAST

Swelling of the breasts with sexual excitement decreases as women get older. By the age of 50, only about one in five women experiences a similar increase in breast size to when they were younger. As a general rule, the more pendulous and slack the breasts – no matter what the woman's age – the less they increase in size with sexual excitement, and this is particularly so in post-menopausal women. With aging comes a significant loss of elasticity in breast tissue, and as hormone levels plummet, there is also a loss of breast tissue and a corresponding reduction in blood vessels. This accounts for the lack of breast swelling during sexual arousal in older women. The areolae continue to become engorged late in the excitement stage and early in the plateau phase, although this frequently occurs in one breast only in older women. (This phenomenon is rarely seen in younger women.) Women over 50 may retain nipple erection for hours after an orgasm.

While the sexual flush occurs in three-quarters of all women under the age of 40, it occurs much less frequently in older women, affecting only about half. By the age of 60, however, only in about one in eight women experiences such flushes. After the age of 60, it seems to disappear altogether, unless a woman is taking hormone replacement therapy. When the flush does appear, it spreads in exactly the same sequence as in a younger woman, though it may be less widespread on the thighs, buttocks, and back. In older women, then, the sexual flush usually appears only on the abdomen, chest, neck, and face.

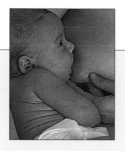

CHAPTER FIVE

THE NURTURING BREAST

The main physiological role of the breast
is to provide nourishment for babies
through the production of milk. Much of
the lifelong bond that a woman forms
with her children may originate in the
pleasure breastfeeding gives. Both mother
and baby derive comfort and closeness
from this intimate contact.

WHY BREASTFEEDING?

A woman's right to choose should extend through all the options available in pregnancy, childbirth, and beyond, and this is also the case for infant feeding from the breast or bottle. But the choice between breast- and bottlefeeding is not simply a matter of deciding the most convenient of two equally good alternatives; all the evidence shows that breastfeeding is better for a variety of reasons. It must be said, however, that if you choose to bottlefeed your baby you are by no means a failed mother. Neither will your baby come to harm if you are aware of the differences between breastfeeding and bottlefeeding and take practical steps to compensate for them. Let me run through the most important things for you to think about.

THE PERFECT MIXTURE AND THE PERFECT DISPENSER

Once you become pregnant, your body gears up to feed your newborn baby, and it comes up with the perfect formula. Your milk contains everything your baby needs, and it is always at the right temperature. In addition, breast milk is always sterile and confers on your baby immunity to certain infections – something that formula cannot do.

When you offer your baby your breast, you are not simply offering him nourishment but also warmth, safety, and the skin-to-skin contact that the process of evolution has led your baby to want and love. The way in which we experience satisfaction and love in infancy has a great deal to do with the degree to which we are able to give and experience these things as adults.

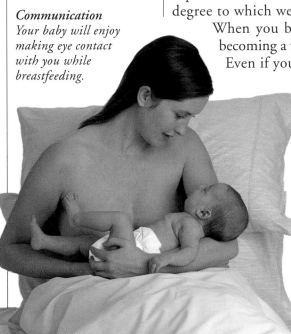

Communication
Your baby will enjoy making eye contact with you while breastfeeding.

When you breastfeed your baby, you give him a head start in his becoming a warm and accepting individual.

Even if you bottlefeed your baby, you don't have to deny him the same sort of skin-to-skin contact achieved through breastfeeding. You can undo your clothes and nestle your baby at the breast when you give him a bottle – and so can your partner.

EARLY COMMUNICATION

For most of the time when she is being breastfed, a baby looks into her mother's face and makes eye contact with her. Although a baby learns her mother's smell and the sound of her voice very quickly after birth, it is through breastfeeding that she begins to recognize her mother's face and also learns how satisfying it is to make eye contact as a means of communication.

If you bottlefeed your baby, don't encourage her to hold her bottle and feed herself as soon as she can; this robs her of the great satisfaction of being fed and looked at by you.

THE TIME FACTOR

Milk from a bottle comes out more quickly and with less effort than from a breast. Most babies are able to finish a bottle feed in a few minutes, especially after they are a month or two old. An eight- or ten-week-old breastfed baby, however, spends about 20 minutes on each breast five times a day – even if much of this time is devoted to comfort sucking rather than active feeding. For a breastfed baby, this adds up to over three hours out of every 24 being held close to her mother and feeling happy and secure, and this is apart from the time that her mother spends playing with her, talking to her, stimulating her interest, and amusing her. If you are going to bottlefeed your baby, it really is important that you give some thought to how you can compensate for the one-to-one time that a breastfed baby has with her mother just by virtue of being breast- rather than bottlefed.

BETTER FOR MOTHER

Many women find breastfeeding not only satisfying but intensely pleasurable. This may be the deciding factor that makes some mothers persevere in the face of sore nipples, inconvenience, and even requests from their partners to bottlefeed rather than breastfeed (see p.84). Breastfeeding undoubtedly gives some women what can only be described as erotic sensations, but of a more serene nature than they have previously experienced. Apart from the consideration of giving your breastfed baby a start in life that cannot be bettered, think hard before you cut yourself off from these deep satisfactions.

A MOTHER'S MILK

All mothers are anatomically equipped to feed their babies – even more than one baby, as with twins. There is no such thing as a mother physically incapable of feeding her baby, except in some cases of breast surgery. Breast milk is a baby's natural food, and he will not reject it; there is no such thing as a mother's milk that does not suit her baby.

If your milk is slow to come at first, it is just a matter of time and practice before the supply becomes established. Remember, it is the amount of fatty tissue in the breasts that largely determines their size, but it is the glands deep in the breast that do the work of producing milk. You don't have to worry if your breasts are small – it's not breast size, but how much your baby takes that affects milk production. If a baby's appetite is not very great he will not suck very often and his mother's breasts will not produce very much milk. If, however, a baby sucks often and feeds eagerly, his mother's breasts will respond to this frequent stimulation by producing more milk.

Milk supply will fluctuate throughout the whole time that a mother is breastfeeding because a baby's appetite is never constant. Even half an hour after a feed, the mother's breasts will contain some milk. If feeding becomes less frequent, the breasts will produce less. For example, a woman who returns to work when her baby is a few months old, so that the baby is being bottle- or spoonfed during the day, will probably find that she can still produce enough milk for an early morning and an evening feed. It is not a good idea to interrupt breastfeeding in the early stages of lactation as this inhibits the milk flow and prevents the establishment of a healthy pattern. Once the baby is older she will not feed so often and the supply will reduce accordingly.

INSUFFICIENT MILK SYNDROME

From about the mid-1970s onward, professionals working with mothers and babies began to take note of the increasing frequency with which women cited insufficient milk as a reason not to breastfeed their babies at all, or to do so for only a very short time. This finding was labeled insufficient milk syndrome (IMS), and it has been identified in many corners of the world. Researchers have generally concluded that IMS is the result of cultural factors rather than the waning of women's physical ability to produce sufficient milk.

Causes Researchers cite the following factors in causing IMS: the pressures of modern urban life; the aggressive promotion of powdered milk, which convinces some women that their own milk is not sufficiently nutritious; unnecessary supplementary bottlefeeding; the practice of hospitals and clinics giving mothers free samples of infant formula supplied by powdered milk companies; the lack of support for breastfeeding from mothers' partners; and the snowballing effect of fewer women being familiar with breastfeeding techniques because they have not witnessed them at home when they were growing up. All of these things militate against relaxed, assured breastfeeding and a mother's confidence in an ample milk supply. The practice of scheduled feedings also aggravates IMS, because the baby is not allowed to regulate her own milk supply naturally by sucking on demand. This situation worsens if women try to ensure that they have "full breasts" by lengthening the time between feeds – the very thing that is calculated to decrease milk production.

MEN'S FEELINGS ABOUT BREASTFEEDING

Everyone writing about breastfeeding stresses how important it is for a woman's partner to be supportive. A woman's psychological state can affect her milk production, and if a man constantly discourages his partner from breastfeeding or even nags her to stop it is possible that this negative attitude will cause an impeded milk flow. Since breastfeeding is so important to infants, and since women are endowed by nature to do so, why, then, are some men opposed to their partners' breastfeeding their babies?

One of the reasons is simple jealousy; the baby at the breast can be seen (consciously or otherwise) as a competitor for the mother's affection or an obstacle between her and her partner. The more familiar a man is with the sight of women breastfeeding their babies, the more likely he is to accept it as part of the natural order. But few of us do see babies being breastfed anymore, even in the home; breastfeeding is often done out of the sight of male members of the family – even quite young children. This is a very unhealthy state of affairs, because it gives children and adolescents quite the wrong messages about breastfeeding. Apparently it is something that should not be done in front of children, even when these same children are exposed every day to sex and violence in newspapers, television programs, and videos.

Another male reaction to women breastfeeding their babies is the suspicion that mother and child are indulging in a sexual activity. This is not so outlandish as it appears at first. In our culture the breast is seen as having a primarily sexual significance: the large-breasted women with manufactured cleavages that we see so often in the media are not inviting admiration for their breastfeeding capacity. Of course the breast has a sexual significance (see p.72), which is just as natural as its feeding function, and some women do experience a quasi-sexual pleasure in breastfeeding. It would be profoundly unnatural, however, to allow one to obliterate the other, or to suppose that the two are mutually exclusive.

Some men, initially supportive about a partner's plans to breastfeed, find that in the end they cannot deal with the breasts' new dual role. These men may continue to be tolerant of breastfeeding, but may feel uncomfortable about sexual foreplay involving the breasts, particularly if they have been used to kissing or sucking their partners' nipples before their babies' birth.

Another obstacle to breastfeeding is the refusal of some men to share the marital bed with their babies. It is the most natural thing in the world for a woman to bring her baby into bed to breastfeed at night, but in some cases her partner may consider this an intrusion into what he sees as territory meant only for him and his partner. The reason usually given for this reluctance is that breastfeeding in bed disturbs his sleep. (Incidentally, if you are worried about how safe your baby might be if you bring him into bed, where he and you might fall asleep, try to recall the last time you heard of an authenticated case of a baby being smothered while asleep with his parents.)

INVOLVING YOUR PARTNER

There certainly are men who would like their babies to be bottlefed from as early as possible so that they can also take part in what is, after all, a very satisfying activity. Giving supplementary bottle feeds, however, is not the way to accommodate this altogether natural desire, because it will have an effect on the mother's milk supply. A father may therefore have to wait until his baby is taking some form of solid food before he can join in with feeding. Inviting him to participate in some diaper changing is one possible and tempting answer, although bathing and dressing the baby come closer to the mark. A pleasant way to breastfeed your baby is to sit or lie in close physical contact with your partner so that the feeding really becomes an activity for three.

Family feeding
Let your partner experience the joys of breastfeeding by encouraging his close physical contact with you and the baby.

BREAST VERSUS BOTTLE

Despite the convenience, suitability, and desirability of breast milk, the practice of bottlefeeding has taken hold to a greater or lesser extent in almost every human settlement that can be reached by a truck. There is no evidence, however, that women of any race or ethnic group produce more or less milk than others, while there is plenty of evidence that, before the notion of feeding babies by the clock, insufficiency of milk was virtually unknown. The notion of scheduled feedings was soon followed by the advent of the bottle and the export of artificial feeding methods from the U.S. and Europe to parts of the world where insufficiency of milk was rare.

SCHEDULED FEEDINGS

The essentially bizarre idea that babies, with all their differences in weight, appetite, and temperament, should be fed at the same regular intervals and that to feed them on demand is somehow "spoiling" them became prevalent in Western hospitals in the nineteenth century. Not surprisingly, these places were run by male doctors, few of whom knew much about breastfeeding. In the mid-1850s, Florence Nightingale's reorganization of nursing made hospital routines and practices more systematized. Much of this was a real improvement, but regular routines imposed on new mothers in hospitals only served to increase the difficulties of breastfeeding, thus hastening its decline. The result was generations of women with engorged breasts, aching nipples, and sodden clothes, not to mention hungry, tearful, and frustrated babies.

Since the way our needs are met in infancy can have a significant effect on the way we try to satisfy them in later life, screaming for nourishment, often for long periods, cannot be a sound basis for character development, let alone a healthy attitude to food. What could be more likely to spoil a baby's character than teaching him that he has to scream for food and attention?

Given the problems breastfeeding mothers had with scheduled feedings, it is not surprising that many jumped to take advantage of formula milks. This happened at the end of the nineteenth century, when a process was developed that converted cows' milk to a form that could be tolerated by the infant stomach. Of course, bottlefeeding by the clock is no more satisfactory for babies than strictly regulated breastfeeding, but at least it does not actually decrease the milk supply. If a woman is persuaded that feeding her baby at regular intervals is the only course, the bottle must seem to be the obvious vehicle for doing it. The pressure to abandon the breast and take to the bottle was and is, in all cases, social rather than physiological.

THE UBIQUITOUS BOTTLE

There cannot be many places more remote from outside influences than an isolated, rural region of Yemen. Yet a recent study found that an increasing level of bottlefeeding was an important factor in the inadequate nutrition of young Yemenis. In such areas, poverty often leads women to overdilute the

Feeding my daughter Emily on demand caused countless arguments with my mother, who belongs to the generation that believed in feeding every four hours on the hour. That approach just turns feeding into a battle of wills, which seems all wrong to me.

ALISON, 29, DOCTOR

formula, causing their babies to become undernourished. Bottlefeeding can also be harmful to the health of babies in any region where supplies of fresh water are limited. Without a ready supply of clean water and fuel, sterilization procedures are often badly followed, and babies are then open to infections, which can prove dangerous, if not fatal.

Many mothers who bottlefeed in developing countries do so because they believe that formula provides better nourishment for their children than breast milk. The lure of modernity is hard to resist. It is ironic that companies spend huge sums on research to try to reproduce breast milk as exactly as possible, while mothers who can ill afford it feed formula to their babies, even though they themselves have quantities of the genuine article. Once their own mik has dried up they are left with no alternative to the bottle.

The one vital ingredient that a powdered-milk company cannot include in its formula is the immunity from certain diseases that the antibodies in breast milk confer on babies. This missing ingredient is all the more crucial where primary medical care is uncertain and infant mortality is already high. If the added value carried by breast milk was clearly understood, far fewer women in the Third World would switch from breast to bottle.

FEEDING CHOICES IN THE DEVELOPED WORLD

There is no clear answer as to why women in the developed world have gone over in such droves to bottlefeeding, though research that has been carried out in connection with ethnic groups in multicultural societies does offer some clues. A recent inquiry in Texas into the proportion of women who start their newborn babies on the breast found that only 45 percent of Anglo-American women, 27 percent of Mexican-American women, and 14 percent of African-American women did so. The central factor here appeared not to be ethnic origins as such but the woman's level of education: whatever her ethnic origin, the better educated a woman was, the greater the likelihood that she would start her baby on the breast. At the same time, an inquiry into the decline in breastfeeding in Sheffield, England, came up with similar findings. Those mothers who had continued in education past the age of 18 were more likely to start their babies on the breast than those who had not. Breastfeeding in general had increased steadily throughout the 1970s but had begun to fall rapidly and progressively in the mid-1980s.

This last study also highlighted the fact that the number of Asian mothers who were bottlefeeding was rising rapidly. This may be explained to some extent in those first-generation immigrant mothers by language problems in hospitals. Many Sikh and Hindu women don't put their babies to their breasts until the colostrum is exhausted, since they think it is harmful. What initially looks like a refusal to breastfeed may be taken by hospital staff as a desire to bottlefeed, and then perhaps the mothers take the path of least resistance. In addition, these religions place certain food prohibitions on lactating women, and a mother might have to prepare special meals for herself in addition to those for her family, which can be arduous.

BREASTFEEDING PRACTICES WORLDWIDE

Throughout the world, a great variety of beliefs and practices relating to breastfeeding exist. Some of them may strike us as odd or even misguided – we can be grateful, for instance, that modern nutritional science can help us avoid erroneous beliefs about a breastfeeding woman's diet. On the other hand, we can learn a great deal from cultures where there is an unbroken tradition of breastfeeding and where women have not learned to feel inhibited and uncertain about feeding their babies.

THE FAMILIAL BREAST

In cultures with a more relaxed attitude to breastfeeding than our own, it is sometimes not a matter of too much concern who feeds the baby. In some African and Asian societies, babies and children have access to any woman who is lactating within the extended family. A moment's thought will show how sensible this is. If a woman is engaged in something that is important to the family but that separates her from her baby, it is altogether wiser that a convenient breast should be offered than that the baby go hungry.

In our society, the fact that a breastfeeding mother has no substitute often helps to push her toward reliance on the bottle. It is notoriously difficult to both hold down a job and breastfeed a baby, and frequently it is just not possible for the household to do without the mother's income, no matter how much she wants to feed her baby herself. Many mothers would not feel

Slings
African women carry their babies in slings that allow them to swing the child easily around to the front for breastfeeding.

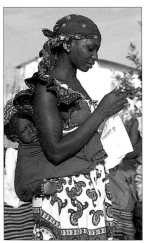

African child-care
It is common for African women to share child-care, and this communal approach can even extend to breastfeeding.

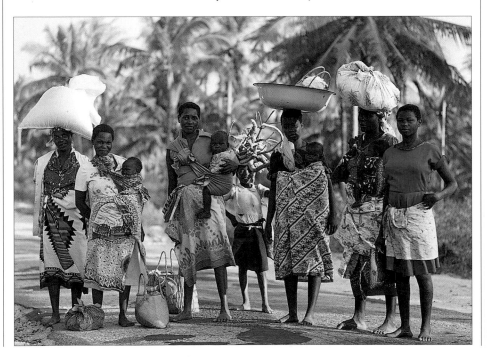

comfortable about letting someone else breastfeed their baby anyway, even if this was on offer. Although the human breast is adaptable enough so that it is quite possible to maintain just a morning and an evening feed, yet not be overflowing in between times, most women seem to feel that it is all or nothing and breastfeed for only a few short months.

THE BREAST AS COMFORTER AND TOY

In virtually all non-industrialized countries, feeding is totally on demand, even around the clock, as babies frequently sleep with their mothers. In such societies, a crying baby must be ministered to immediately. People in these societies regard Europeans, who are prepared to leave their babies to cry, as profoundly lacking in decent human feeling. If, in answer to the suggestion that she suckle the baby, a European mother says that she knows the baby is not hungry, she is regarded as foolish as well. Hungry or not, crying babies need to be comforted, and what is more comforting than to be put to the breast?

It's not uncommon in some cultures for women long past childbearing age to offer their milkless breasts to babies in need of comfort. Examples are also recorded of men putting an unhappy baby to their nipples. In many sub-Saharan African societies, women carry babies on their backs, held in position with lengths of cloth, and it is an easy matter to shift infants to the front and offer them the breast. It is also quite usual to see a young child run back to her mother for a feed and put the breast in her mouth herself.

Where it is commonplace for women to breastfeed in public, everyone is accustomed to the fact that the breast is the baby's first toy. Once the first urgent hunger has been relieved, the growing baby practices her newfound skills. She prods and pokes her mother's flesh or holds one breast while she sucks the other – very much as a puppy or a kitten will knead its mother's breasts. The mother flips her nipple gently in and out of the baby's mouth and the baby smiles and chuckles. Because of the more rigid attitudes toward breastfeeding that are still prevalent in our culture, such pleasantries are generally confined to the privacy of the home and, even there, possibly out of sight of others. It is little wonder that young people have begun to think that breastfeeding is something slightly shameful, and that it is only to be practiced in total seclusion.

BREASTFEEDING AS A CONTRACEPTIVE

Worldwide there is a belief that the breastfeeding of one child can help to prevent the conception of another. Although this belief is based on accurate observation, it is not completely reliable. It is a fact that the hormone that promotes lactation inhibits

PAYMENT FOR BREASTFEEDING

Breastfeeding for pay by someone who is not the baby's mother, called the wet-nurse (see p.24), was well known in historical times. The idea of the mother herself receiving payment is less familiar but, according to Islamic rule, a woman may demand payment from her husband for breastfeeding. If another woman is willing to feed the baby voluntarily, however, and is acceptable to the father, no payment will be made to the wife. If the mother does not wish to feed the child, even if paid, she has no obligation to do so. It's likely that, in a fiercely patriarchal culture, this custom has more to do with a father's "ownership" of his child than with the issue of breastfeeding; traditionally most women fed their own babies.

ovulation, and breastfeeding women are therefore less likely to conceive than others. Ovulation escape does occur, however, and while breastfeeding may help to maintain an interval of two or three years between pregnancies in conditions where the infants are almost totally dependent on suckling for nourishment, it is not a foolproof means of contraception and should never be relied on (see p.94). Nevertheless, it is quite probable that breastfeeding is sometimes prolonged by a mother in the hope that it will prevent her from becoming pregnant again too quickly.

WITHDRAWAL OF MILK AND MALNUTRITION

The disease of malnutrition referred to as *kwashiorkor*, which is characterized by a distended stomach, listlessness, and lightening of the hair, was first documented in Ghana. The literal meaning of *kwashiorkor* is "heat," and it is the term used by the women whose children were being studied. They had observed that their children became prey to the disease when the arrival of a new baby either prevented them from being breastfed or drastically cut down their supply of milk. It was thought that the newborn child directed feelings of jealousy, or "heat," towards the older child already suckling from the mother's breast. This is a good example of accurate observation followed by a mistaken conclusion. The older child *did* suffer from the coming of the baby, not because of any malign influence but because of protein deprivation when the milk was withdrawn.

BREASTFEEDING PROHIBITIONS

In many societies there are rules or taboos that apply to breastfeeding women. The two main categories of behavior they relate to are sexual relations and food. Most of these prohibitions are intended to protect the baby, though occasionally they are for the benefit of the mother or even the father.

SEXUAL PROHIBITIONS

Some societies believe that semen can contaminate breast milk. A man who believes this may spur his wife on to bottlefeed rather than abstain from sex. Others think of women as being ritually unclean after the birth of a child. This state is not usually thought to last more than a few weeks or months, but in some cases sex is prohibited until lactation is finished, and again this will act as a spur to male intervention.

Exclusively female fluids – menstrual blood and breast milk – are thought to be dangerous to adult males in some cultures. After giving birth, a woman is bleeding from the vagina and lactating; sexual contact with her is therefore thought to be doubly dangerous.

Where prolonged periods of sexual abstinence after childbirth exist, these may well have originated to protect the baby's food source. If babies are totally dependent on the breast for nourishment, it is necessary to put off the birth of the next child until the older sibling can do without breast milk. The practice of weaning one child while feeding another, however, is not uncommon.

FOOD PROHIBITIONS

In cultures where certain foods are thought to have significant properties apart from their nutritional value, pregnancy, birth, and suckling are frequently surrounded by food taboos. Some of these have no nutritional basis and may be detrimental to the health of the mother, the child, or both. If, for example, high-protein foods such as meat are denied to a pregnant or lactating woman because they are considered too "strong" for her condition, and especially when these foods form a significant part of her normal intake, she may suffer from impoverished nutrition at the very time when a balanced diet is vital to her and her baby. The ability of malnourished women to produce milk of sufficient nutritional value to promote growth in their children is quite astonishing, however (see p.96), so the baby is less likely to lose out.

Worldwide, eggs are both ritually favored and prohibited. They are commonly prohibited to lactating women as they are supposed to be the cause of breathlessness, vomiting, diarrhea, and, in at least one area, baldness in babies at the breast. On the other hand, in many societies eggs are seen as representing fertility and reproduction, and therefore figure prominently as a food item to be eaten by pubescent girls.

"Hot" and "cold" foods In many societies in India, South America, and Africa, foods fall into two main categories: hot and cold. These do not relate to whether or not the food has been cooked or heated, but to what is thought to be the essence of the food. The division is similar to the Chinese concept of *yin* and *yang,* which is also applied to foods: "cold" corresponds to *yin* and "hot" to *yang.* The boundaries may differ from one society to the next, but fruit and vegetables are almost everywhere thought to be "cold."

"Cold" foods are commonly avoided after giving birth. Communities in Malaysia, for example, prohibit all fruits (except cooked bananas), vegetables, fried foods, and many kinds of fish for 40 days after the birth, as well as tea, which is "cold" (coffee is "hot"). The mother's diet consists mainly of rice and certain kinds of roasted fish, which means that mother and baby will be deficient in calcium, some B vitamins, and vitamins A and C.

The prohibition of "cold" foods is thought to "dry up" the blood flow after birth and to help reduce the swollen tissues; this is considered to be best achieved by eating only "hot" foods. During the 40-day prohibition period, the mother also uses a "roasting bed," underneath which burning coals are placed, and she periodically holds a wrapped, heated stone on her abdomen to aid in shrinking the swollen tissues. Interestingly, a woman in this community who is receiving medication from a doctor or the local clinic is exempt from the food prohibitions, because the medicine is considered to be "hot" enough to combat the "cold" elements in the normal diet.

The women of the Malaysian community consider that all the forbidden foods transmit toxins to babies even though they are all freely eaten during pregnancy. This is an example of how purely cultural beliefs and practices can affect the nutritional content of breast milk.

THE PHYSICAL PROCESS

Breast changes are one of the earliest signs of pregnancy and result from the secretion of the pregnancy hormone progesterone. Two early signs are swelling of the areola and, shortly after, rapid swelling of the breasts themselves. Almost all pregnant women experience tenderness down the sides of their breasts and tingling and soreness of their nipples. This is due to the considerable growth of the milk duct system and the formation of many more lobules. The lobules are made up of little sacs called alveoli, consisting of clusters of glandular cells enclosing a small space; these expand, and secretions gather inside them. The increase in breast size is due to the expansion and multiplication of the alveoli and their ducts.

Another diagnostic sign of pregnancy is the increasingly visible blood vessels on the skin of the breasts. This is due to the blood vessels that supply the breast expanding and filling with blood. The nipples and areolae become darker in color. Even before you miss your first period, your nipples will feel bruised and your breasts may feel heavy and tender and could be measurably larger. The little bumps on the areola, the tubercles of Montgomery, enlarge and become more prominent; they keep the nipple lubricated and protected during pregnancy and breastfeeding. The nipples become less firmly bound to the underlying breast tissue, making them more mobile and easier for the suckling infant to take in his mouth.

MILK PRODUCTION BEGINS

The development of the glands and ducts during pregnancy is an extension of the growth that follows puberty; as in puberty (see p.41), estrogen is primarily responsible for the growth of the ducts, and progesterone for the growth of the glandular buds, and, as before, these ovarian hormones require the presence of both follicle-stimulating hormone (FSH) and luteinizing hormone (LH), both of which are secreted by the pituitary gland in the brain, to exert their full effect.

The structure of the lactating breast depends on the amount of milk it contains, but in general as the lobules enlarge, they compress the walls that separate them. The cells lining the alveoli accumulate fat droplets and small granules of protein – the basic components of milk. By a process of apocrine secretion (similar to that of sweat), these fat droplets and protein granules are released into the alveolar sacs. The surfaces of the alveoli become irregular, and as the secretions accumulate they swell and flatten. By the fifth or sixth month of pregnancy, the breasts are usually fully capable of producing milk.

HORMONES AND MILK PRODUCTION

Prolactin, produced by the pituitary gland in the brain, is essential to milk production. It aids the action of progesterone and estrogen, but can also produce mammary growth. Many other hormones are involved in successful milk production, including steroid hormones from the adrenal glands, and

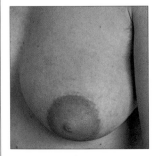

Changes in pregnancy
During pregnancy the blood vessels of the breasts are more prominent, seen as blue lines across the breast. The areolae enlarge and darken.

thyroid hormone. A hormone from the placenta, human placental lactogen (HPL), also plays an important part in the development of the mammary glands during pregnancy. HPL, structurally very similar to the growth hormone produced by the pituitary gland, is produced in large amounts – 1 to 2 grams daily – in late pregnancy, a time when the breasts are preparing for maximum milk production. Estrogen inhibits milk production during pregnancy; after childbirth, however, milk production quickly speeds up.

WHEN MILK APPEARS

From about the sixth month of pregnancy onward, the nipples may leak small quantities of a straw-colored fluid called colostrum. Colostrum forms a baby's first food, and production continues for the first two or three days after a baby is born. Colostrum differs from milk – it has a high fat and protein content – and is perfectly suited to a baby's first days of life, when her primitive digestive system is learning to cope with food taken by mouth.

Milk secretion commonly starts on the third day after birth when the milk is said to "come in," and gradually increases to a rate of about 850 milliliters per day (approximately $1\frac{1}{2}$ pints), although yields as high as 3 liters a day ($5\frac{1}{4}$ pints) have been recorded. Interestingly, fluid intake appears to have little effect on milk production, so there's no need to drink vast quantities of water when you are breastfeeding — though nursing mothers often do get thirsty.

THE "LET-DOWN" REFLEX

The milk in a mother's breasts is not available for her baby until it has been ejected (let down) from the milk glands. For breastfeeding to go smoothly, therefore, regular let-down is essential. The ejection of milk is stimulated by several factors, the strongest being the sensation of the baby sucking at the nipple, but some mothers find that hearing the baby's cry or even thinking about feeding him makes her milk flow. Such is the power of the let-down reflex that milk has been known to shoot from the nipples of a nursing mother over a meter (3 feet) across the room when she hears her baby's hungry cry.

The let-down of the breast milk depends on nerves carrying messages to the brain that milk is needed, and a chemical messenger, the hormone oxytocin, from the brain to the breast to release the milk from the glands down to the nipples. (It is worth noting here that a nipple with its nerve supply intact is a crucial part of the reflex arc that brings about let-down. If the nipple has lost its nerve supply, which might happen in the case of plastic surgery, particularly in a breast reduction operation, then the let-down reflex cannot occur, and breastfeeding will not be possible.)

CHANGES IN BREAST PIGMENTATION

Melanocytes are skin cells that contain melanin, the pigment that controls the color of the skin and makes the skin go brown when it is exposed to ultraviolet rays from the sun. They are found in large numbers in the nipple and areola. Melanocyte-stimulating hormone (MSH) is produced increasingly as pregnancy progresses, and accounts for the darkening of the nipple and areola. A woman's nipple and areola deepen in color according to her skin type – the darker the skin, the deeper the color of the nipple – and the changed pigmentation will then become permanent.

THE LET-DOWN REFLEX

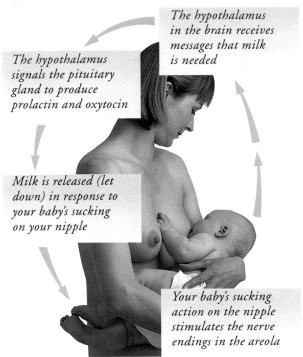

The hypothalamus in the brain receives messages that milk is needed

The hypothalamus signals the pituitary gland to produce prolactin and oxytocin

Milk is released (let down) in response to your baby's sucking on your nipple

Your baby's sucking action on the nipple stimulates the nerve endings in the areola

Lactation is controlled by the hormone prolactin, which is responsible for the production of milk, and oxytocin, which forces milk from the glands into the ducts.

Oxytocin causes the cells that surround the alveoli to contract, thus forcing milk out of them and into the ducts. During suckling oxytocin continues to be released, and this can commonly cause uterine contractions, which a mother may notice and even find painful while breastfeeding.

The cerebral cortex, the part of the brain that is responsible for emotional and intellectual processes, has an important overriding influence on all these mechanisms, and so, not surprisingly, lactation can be profoundly influenced by a woman's emotions and psychological state.

OVULATION DURING BREASTFEEDING

Under normal conditions lactation continues for as long as suckling goes on. Breastfeeding in Western countries is usually practiced for only a few months after birth, but in some African and Asian countries lactation may continue for as long as two or three years (see p.89). Even until the eighteenth or nineteenth century this was also the case in Britain, especially among poorer women.

The inhibition of ovulation after giving birth is probably due to the suppression of luteinizing hormone (LH) and follicle-stimulating hormone (FSH) by the lactation hormones prolactin and oxytocin. This makes lactation a time of relative infertility – that is, a woman is less fertile than usual when breastfeeding, but this doesn't mean she can't conceive. As soon as sex is resumed, all couples must begin to take precautions whether the mother is breastfeeding or not. If conception does occur during lactation, milk production will continue during the new pregnancy, although the quantity and quality will decrease. You should never rely on lactation as a foolproof method of contraception.

MILK COMPOSITION

The main constituents of breast milk are those that form the basis of all foods: water, carbohydrate, fat, and protein. Water is responsible for transporting nutrients throughout the body, acts as a lubricant and a cushion, and helps to maintain body temperature.

Carbohydrates are broken down to glucose by the body to provide energy. Lactose, an easily digestible sugar, is the main carbohydrate in breast milk; it starts to be produced by the breasts in early pregnancy and can be detected in the mother's blood and urine. Fats provide energy reserves, make us feel full after a meal, carry fat-soluble nutrients, insulate the body, and provide the main material for cell membranes. The fats in breast milk are triglycerides – the commonest form of fat in foods – and are manufactured from circulating fatty acids in the breast itself. Proteins support the growth and maintenance of the body, regulate the action of hormones, form antibodies, and serve as the building material for skin, muscles, organs, and bones. Milk proteins – the most distinctive being lactalbumin – are probably synthesized by cells in the milk glands from amino acids circulating in the body, although some plasma proteins also appear in milk.

BREAST MILK AND COWS' MILK

Although cows' milk has similar constituents to breast milk, it is unsuitable for young babies in its raw state because the proportions are quite different: in untreated cows' milk, the protein content is much higher, while the level of carbohydrates is too low. It also contains too high a concentration of minerals for a baby's immature kidneys to handle.

Another important difference is the type of protein in the milks. Most of the protein in cows' milk is casein, which comes from the curds. Most of the protein in breast milk comes from the whey, a more digestible type of protein. Formula milks that are advertised as being very similar to breast milk contain mostly whey proteins; those advertised as being suitable for older or hungrier babies contain mostly casein.

The fat content of human milk may vary from 1 to over 6 grams per 100 milliliters (the average figure is about 4 grams); for instance, foremilk, the watery, thirst-quenching liquid that is released at the beginning of a feed, contains less fat than hindmilk, the thicker, nutritious milk of the main part of a feed. The fat content will also vary depending on the age of the baby. Variation in the milk's fat content is not dependent on racial or ethnic origin. The fat content of cows' milk is comparable, though less variable. The levels of some other nutrients, notably the water-soluble vitamins (that is, vitamin C, which protects against infection, and the B vitamins, which help the body to build proteins and use energy efficiently), change significantly with variations in the mother's diet, so every breastfeeding mother must take care with her daily food intake (see p.96) to ensure that she remains well nourished.

VITAMINS AND MINERALS

One important feature of breast milk is the ratio of calcium to phosphorus. Calcium is an important ingredient of bones and teeth, and is involved in the action of the muscles and nerves, blood clotting, and the immune system. Phosphorus is present with calcium in the bones and teeth, and also plays an important role in the genetic material of cells and cell membranes.

Ideally, for calcium to be absorbed properly, there needs to be twice as much calcium as phosphorus, and this is the case with breast milk. Other vitamins and minerals in the milk are present in an easily absorbed form. Although formula appears to contain larger amounts of these nutrients, they are not completely absorbed, so formula is not actually more nutritious. Breast milk is low in iron, which is crucial to the transport of oxygen in the blood, but newborn babies have a supply of iron in their bodies that will last several months, so there is no real need for the iron supplements that are added to formula milk. By the time a baby's initial supply runs out, she will be on solid food and will be able to get iron from a varied diet. Although it was once thought that breast milk is low in vitamin D, it has been found to be present in a water-soluble form (vitamin D is usually fat-soluble). This vitamin can be manufactured by the body in response to sunlight, but in rare cases a baby may need vitamin D supplements – low-birth-weight babies, for example, or those who do not get enough sunlight. If you are concerned, consult your doctor, who will be able to advise you.

One of the most remarkable features of breast milk is the way it adapts to the baby's changing needs. The milk a mother produces when her baby is six months old will be different from what she produced when the baby was born: more thirst-quenching, and lower in fat and protein.

DIET AND BREAST MILK

Another property of breast milk is that, apart from the factors mentioned below, diet has relatively little influence on milk yield or composition, and established lactation is surprisingly little affected by short periods of severe deprivation. Mothers who are suffering from malnutrition continue to be able to provide nourishment for their babies long after one would expect this to be the case. A woman's physical resources are marshalled by her body to promote the well-being of her baby, at whatever cost to herself.

This is not a state of affairs to be recommended, however. While no special diet is necessary for a nursing mother, she does need adequate nutrition, and this means taking in extra calories as long as she is breastfeeding.

THE ENERGY COSTS OF MILK PRODUCTION

The fuel for milk production can come from maternal food intake, stored energy sources (usually body fat), or a combination of the two. A baby may require about 1¾ pints (850 milliliters) of milk a day, which provides him with 68 calories per 100 milliliters, or 578 calories daily. Milk production is only about 90 percent efficient, so a woman requires an extra 700 calories a day when feeding is at its peak. This should come mostly from increased dietary intake; the remainder can be taken from fat stores laid down in pregnancy. Weight loss of more than 1 pound (0.5 kg) a week can inhibit milk supply.

AN ADEQUATE DIET

Although a nursing mother needs some extra calories, she also needs plenty of nutrients. There is no room in her diet for "empty calories" – that is, foods high in unnecessary fats and sugars but containing few other nutrients. The additional calories are best taken from extra servings of fruit, vegetables, meat or meat alternatives (beans or lentils, for example), and breads. Nutritional requirements for breastfeeding mothers are higher than during pregnancy.

VITAMIN A	VITAMIN C	VITAMIN E	ZINC
Sources *Carrots, beef liver, spinach, sweet potato, milk, cheese, and apricots. Bright orange and dark green vegetables are rich in beta-carotene, a form of vitamin A*	**Sources** *Red and green peppers, tomatoes, broccoli, brussels sprouts, blackcurrants, strawberries, oranges, lemons, grapefruit, and cantaloupe melons*	**Sources** *Polyunsaturated oils, particularly wheatgerm oil and soybean oil, whole grains, nuts, and seeds, especially sunflower seeds*	**Sources** *Meat, shellfish, poultry, peas, black beans, and yogurt*
Function *A most versatile vitamin, vitamin A is active throughout the body, and plays an important role in maintaining body linings and skin, the immune system, cell development, growth (particularly growth of bone and teeth), vision, and reproduction*	**Function** *Essential to the production of collagen, which is a protein that forms the basis for bones, teeth, skin, connective tissue, tendons, and scar tissue. Vitamin C supports the immune system, protects against infection, and helps the body absorb iron from food*	**Function** *Protects blood and lung cells from the possible harmful effects of oxygen, which could destroy the cell membranes by a process called oxidation*	**Function** *Assists enzymes in cells throughout the body, boosts the immune system, and is essential to wound healing, sperm production, fetal development, and growth in children; also important to normal taste perception and vision*

A woman needs only slightly more protein, but significantly greater amounts of vitamins A, C, and E, and zinc. Iron and folic acid intake, which need to be very high during pregnancy, now return to normal levels. Some foods that can help boost vitamin intake are shown in the chart above.

DIETARY CONTAMINANTS IN BREAST MILK

Most substances that are dissolved in a mother's blood will appear in small amounts in breast milk; these include such drugs as caffeine, alcohol, antibiotics, and barbiturates. A breastfeeding mother should limit her alcohol intake to the occasional single drink, but even this amount may affect the taste of her milk so that her baby finds it unpleasant and drinks less than normal. Caffeine may make a baby jumpy and wakeful. Some foods, such as onions or garlic, may affect the taste of milk, causing the baby discomfort; careful observation will help avoid this.

ILLNESS, DRUGS, AND BREAST MILK

If a breastfeeding mother becomes ill with the common cold or flu, the only reason not to breastfeed is if she feels too ill to do so. A mother and her baby are constantly in close contact, so the baby is quite likely to pick up the infection anyway; there's no point in depriving him of breast milk. If the mother is confined to bed and feels very weak and tired, she can still express her milk so that her partner or a friend can feed the baby; otherwise the baby will have to take formula milk until the mother can breastfeed again. (A supply of frozen expressed milk will be useful in this situation.) A mother with a serious communicable illness such as tuberculosis or hepatitis will have to be separated from her baby, but even in this case the baby can be fed her

Vitamin and mineral sources
A breastfeeding mother needs enough nutrients from her diet for herself and her baby. The chart above suggests sources for vitamins A, C, and E, and zinc, which are particularly important at this time.

mother's expressed milk. A hospital stay needn't mean that breastfeeding has to stop; the mother can make special arrangements with the nursing staff in order to continue. A general anaesthetic may preclude breastfeeding, however, as it will persist in the body for a while and will also cause grogginess. It's a good idea, therefore, to express and freeze milk in advance, if possible, so that someone at home can continue to feed it to the baby in your absence. In this way, the baby will not miss out on the nutrients in breast milk, even if she misses the pleasure of feeding from her mother. Local anaesthetics containing lignocaine or bupivacaine, which may sometimes be administered during labor, are quite safe.

Diabetes In many cases breastfeeding can actually be very beneficial to a mother with diabetes as it may reduce her need for insulin. In the first few days after birth, the baby's blood sugar must be closely monitored until glucose levels stabilize. The mother's glucose level, insulin dose, and calorie requirements must also be carefully monitored as long as she is breastfeeding. There is no danger to the baby from the mother's insulin injections, as they serve only to bring her insulin up to a normal level. It is important for a diabetic mother to discuss her medication with her doctor if she is intending to breastfeed. While there are drugs available that are quite safe for breastfeeding, some – such as chlorpropamide – pass into the milk and could cause low blood-sugar levels in the baby.

A diabetic mother must be particularly vigilant in avoiding sore nipples and breast infections (see p.134), and any problems should receive immediate treatment. When the baby is weaned and milk production ceases, the insulin dose and calorie requirements will have to be adjusted again.

Breast lumps Although breast lumps are less likely to be detected because of the many changes occurring in the lactating breast, they can appear during breastfeeding just as at any other time. If a lump is found to be cancerous, there is no risk to the baby, but the mother may have to give up breastfeeding so she can undergo treatment without delay.

AIDS A mother who is HIV-positive (that is, who carries the virus that leads to AIDS) may well pass the virus on to her unborn child. The likelihood of this is somewhere between 20 and 50 percent, according to recent studies. If the baby is born uninfected, the mother should not breastfeed, because HIV appears in breast milk and can be passed on to the baby.

DRUGS

Many prescribed drugs, including some antibiotics, will have no adverse affect on a breastfed baby if they pass into the mother's milk. If a doctor knows a woman is breastfeeding, the prescription can be given accordingly, or the mother advised to suspend breastfeeding temporarily if necessary. When choosing drugs, a number of factors bear consideration.

• The baby's age will affect her ability to metabolize drugs. Premature babies have the least capacity to deal with drugs; a baby several months old will be much less affected.

• The mother's needs must be weighed against the benefits to the baby of breastfeeding. If the mother's health is at serious risk and she must take drugs, breastfeeding need not necessarily cease completely; it can be started again once the mother is well.

• The length of time that the mother will be taking the drugs is significant. A course of antibiotics lasting only a few days may have very little effect on the baby even if they do pass into the milk.

• Current knowledge about the drug must be taken into account. Some drugs have been tried and tested and are known not to have any effect on the baby. With newer drugs, however, the effects may be little understood, or there may be conflicting medical opinion.

• The length of time that drugs remain in the mother's body varies greatly. Some are eliminated from the system after only a few hours; others build up in the body over several days, and these may also accumulate in the baby's body if they get into the mother's milk.

• Only drugs that pass into the bloodstream can get into breast milk, and the administration of a drug will determine this. Injected drugs pass directly into the bloodstream; drugs taken by mouth usually do, except for some stomach medications that work locally in the stomach or intestines. Creams applied to the skin are unlikely to pass into the blood.

Your doctor will take into account the fact that you are breastfeeding before prescribing any drug. Over-the-counter medicines, however, may also contain drugs that could affect your milk – even common painkillers and cold remedies. It's always best, therefore, to consult your doctor or pharmacist before taking any medication while breastfeeding. Don't rely on information that you were given when you had your last baby, or what a friend tells you; drugs are available in many different formulations, and new drugs appear on the market all the time.

Social drugs Since social drugs are not necessary to the mothers' health, and indeed may damage it, it follows that they should not be used while she is breastfeeding. Nicotine appears in breast milk; aside from this, a baby whose mother smokes will suffer harmful effects through passive smoking, and have twice the normal risk of crib death (SIDS), not to mention risks of heart and lung disease. Alcohol also passes into milk, and large amounts can actually make the baby drunk. Even moderate drinking on a daily basis can cause delayed muscle development in the baby. Occasional moderate drinking is probably not harmful, but it's a good idea to wait until the alcohol has been metabolized before feeding – allow one hour per drink.

> *I was surprised when I asked my doctor about drugs and breastfeeding and he mentioned alcohol – I hadn't realized that drinking after the pregnancy could affect my baby.*
> JOAN, 33, HOUSEWIFE

THE RESOURCEFUL BREAST

Some women, faced with real obstacles, feel that the odds are stacked against them and it's not worth the attempt to breastfeed. What is so remarkable about the breast is the way it rises to the occasion and produces milk in copious quantities even in the most unpromising circumstances. If a mother can produce milk, however little, and her baby has a healthy sucking reflex, then she can breastfeed, though patience and perseverance may be required.

TWINS

No woman should worry that she won't have enough milk to feed twins – she will. After all, a twin is small and requires less milk at first than a single baby. As twins grow, their mother's breasts will produce sufficient milk to feed them, so she should be positive from the start and believe in herself. For the first six months the feeding regimen with twins can be critical for the mother, her babies, and her family. The guiding rule is that a mother must do what suits her situation best, and a good approach is to take her lead from her babies.

Two crucial needs are planning and encouragement. Few women have ever seen twins being breastfed, so before the babies arrive it is a good idea for the expectant mother to visit another twin home. A doctor, hospital, or a contact at the local La Leche League (see p.200) may well be able to put you in touch. These visits can be used to watch, take notes, learn techniques and routines, ask questions, and seek solutions to possible problems.

As a general rule, it is more difficult to establish breastfeeding with twins. More twins than single babies are premature, and so they take longer to suck well and to get the milk flowing well. It also requires the skill of a juggler to attach and keep two babies on the breast at once, one on each breast, but it can be done with the aid of a chair with arms and pillows. There are several positions for feeding twins: both in front, with their legs side by side or crossed over each other; with their heads to the front and their legs under their mother's arms; or any combination of these. A mother should try them all and opt for what feels the most comfortable. These early efforts are worthwhile, especially since the mother can produce plenty of milk for two over a period of 12 months.

Twins benefit from all the advantages that apply to single breastfed babies, but the protection against infection that they receive in the first few days is of particular value, since twins are more likely to be vulnerable because of prematurity. In

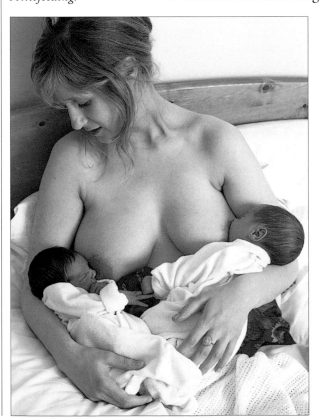

Feeding twins
Breastfeeding your twins enables you to hold and feed both of your babies at the same time, which isn't possible if you are bottlefeeding.

addition, a good deal of money is saved on baby milk. A mother of twins should not set herself unachievable goals; many mothers are happy to partially breastfeed their babies. Relying entirely on breast milk may be unrealistic, because the twins may not have the same feeding and sleeping patterns and their mother may not always have a helper.

THE PREMATURE BABY

A mother who sees her premature baby lying in an incubator and being fed through a tube may feel that she can do nothing to help, and must leave her baby's welfare to the expertise of the hospital staff. While feeding premature babies is never straightforward, breastfeeding is still of particular benefit because of the protection against infection it affords. It is another illustration of the versatility of the breast that the milk from a mother of a premature baby differs from that for a full-term baby; it contains higher levels of protein to give the baby the extra nourishment she needs in the critical first days.

It is therefore worth attempting breastfeeding if at all possible. In this way, however helpless a mother may feel at seeing her tiny baby in an incubator, she will know she has been able to contribute to her well-being.

Newborn premature babies are usually fed intravenously or by stomach tube, so a mother will have to express milk during this time to maintain her supply. This can be difficult, because the events that normally prompt let-down (see p.93) are missing: a baby's hungry cry and the sensation of her sucking at the breast. With persistence, though, it's possible. Expression should be carried out every couple of hours to mimic the frequent feeding of a very small baby. The length of time a mother has to continue expressing will depend on how premature her baby is. Once a baby is strong enough to be taken out of the incubator for short periods, her mother will be able to put her on the breast so both can enjoy close contact and the baby can make her first attempts to suck. Everything may not go smoothly at first. Premature babies need time to learn to latch on, they don't feed very vigorously or for very long, and they often fall asleep at the breast. A baby may need the odd supplementary feed to begin with, and a mother may need to continue expressing to maintain her milk supply until feeding is well established, with the baby latching on successfully and sucking for 15 minutes at a feed.

BREASTFEEDING WITHOUT BREAST MILK

It is a little-known fact that a woman doesn't have to be pregnant to produce breast milk; even a woman who has never carried a child may be able to breastfeed a baby given the constant stimulation of the infant sucking at the breasts. A nursing supplementation device takes advantage of this fact to help adoptive mothers who wish to breastfeed their babies.

The device consists of a plastic pouch or bottle to hold milk or formula and a thin flexible tube that leads from the container to the mother's nipple. The baby sucks at the nipple and receives the milk from the container. The beauty of the system is that the baby's suckling can stimulate the mother's own breast to produce some milk, so although the baby will get milk from only the container at first, eventually he may get some of his mother's own milk as well. The younger the baby, the more likely the system is to be successful.

In a mother who has never been pregnant or lactated before, the breasts won't produce full milk, but the fluid produced will have some nutritional value for the baby. If a woman has breastfed before, or has been pregnant for several months, her breasts will eventually produce full milk. Many mothers will find that they need to continue using the supplementation device for the whole time they're breastfeeding.

Restarting breastfeeding The nursing supplementation device can also be used by women who, for whatever reason, wish to resume breastfeeding after a break. If it is less than a week since lactation stopped (or since the baby was born, if she's never been breastfed), nursing every two hours or so will usually stimulate full milk production in a few days. If it has been more than a week, prolonged use of the nursing supplementation device may be necessary.

BREASTFEEDING AND BREAST SURGERY

Breast surgery can make breastfeeding impossible, depending on the type and the extent of surgery. If the milk ducts are not completely severed from the nipple and some breast tissue remains, there is always the possibility that the breast will be able to produce a little milk. Severing the nerves of the nipple will also interfere with the let-down reflex (see p.93).

Augmentation Implants do not affect a woman's ability to breastfeed unless an incision has been made around the areola. If so, the milk ducts to the nipple may have been cut and milk supply may be poor or nonexistent.

Reduction Whether or not you can breastfeed after reduction surgery will depend on the amount of tissue that has been removed. If the nipples have been relocated then the milk ducts have usually been severed and milk supply is affected. Nevertheless, studies show that about half the women who have had reduction can still breastfeed. If milk supply is reduced, then a nursing supplementation device can be used.

Mastectomy A woman who has had a mastectomy can still feed her baby from the remaining breast. Because one breast is doing all the work, frequent nursing will be necessary at first to build up a good supply. In most cases the mother can eventually provide all the milk her baby needs.

Lumpectomy and radiation therapy A lumpectomy, if it is not very extensive, may not affect a woman's breastfeeding capacity at all, but radiation will. The irradiated breast may not go through the same changes that the normal one does during pregnancy, and it will produce little or no milk. The mother can still feed her baby from the normal breast, however.

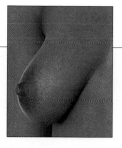

CHAPTER SIX

COSMETIC BREAST SURGERY

The importance of a woman's breasts to her self-image – rightly or wrongly – is reinforced by media images. This has led to a growing acceptance of every woman's right to alter her breasts with cosmetic surgery. All women should be able to receive unbiased, medically sound information about surgery without being made to feel embarrassed or fearful.

DECIDING ON SURGERY

In the developed world, submitting to cosmetic surgery has become an almost inevitable part of getting older among the affluent. The high regard in which youth is held has forced some women to maintain their looks by artificial means. Cosmetic surgery is capable of reversing some of the effects of aging and therefore has flourished because there is a ready market. Not so long ago it was little discussed and almost a taboo subject. Nowadays, women boast about it, and newspapers are happy to report when someone like Betty Ford or Ethel Kennedy is able to change her appearance completely with a face-lift, or the pop singer Cher takes drastic measures and has the last rib removed, the better to define her waistline.

REASONS TO HAVE SURGERY

The results of plastic surgery in many cases are excellent. It's possible for a good surgeon wholly to change the appearance of your breasts and, if you like, the actual contours of your body. Such an operation, however, requires that you be well motivated, because you will inevitably have to bear some form of discomfort and may be somewhat depressed after the procedure until the effects become apparent.

It is very important that you have the operation for the correct reasons and not because a husband, lover, or any third party who is critical of your figure pressures you into undergoing plastic surgery. You will never be happy with the result if this is the case.

If you have serious psychological problems that affect aspects of your life other than your appearance, cosmetic surgery is not going to put them right. If a relationship is disintegrating or a marriage falling apart, plastic surgery isn't going to remedy the situation, and no man will love you more for having a breast uplift. On the other hand, if you have suffered severe psychological stress because of asymmetrical breasts or breasts that are too big, then cosmetic surgery can have long-term benefits that will affect all aspects of your life.

Nowadays, a good reason for having plastic surgery may simply be that your body looks older than you feel; you need seek no further justification. After cosmetic surgery, women are often more at ease with themselves and feel more self-assured; that alone will make them look better.

In the past, women who had plastic surgery to their breasts were usually quite satisfied with the results, partly because they didn't have unrealistic expectations. It's becoming increasingly common, however, for women to seek plastic surgery for breasts with the same idea of unattainable perfection as when they consider a face-lift.

You can have plastic surgery on your breasts at any age, although it is better to wait until your early twenties, when your body has stopped growing. Age is not a deterrent, so at no time do you have to live your life with breasts that make you feel at all uncomfortable. In general, few women regret having had plastic surgery to their breasts, though many regret not doing so.

IF YOU ARE CONTEMPLATING BREAST SURGERY

Cosmetic breast surgery is one area of medicine that has been with us for many years, and plastic surgeons are good at it. Women have undergone breast surgery for almost a hundred years, breast reduction having been known for many decades and breast augmentation for a somewhat shorter time. Experience has shown that surgical operations on the breasts are among the safest in existence. There is, of course, the very small risk that applies to all surgical procedures when a general anesthetic is given, but the risk is from the anesthesia, not the surgical intervention. Most women consider this risk a fair trade-off for the opportunity to change or enhance their appearance or relieve physical discomfort, but it must be borne in mind nonetheless.

CHOOSING A COSMETIC SURGEON

Before you seriously contemplate cosmetic surgery, you should be aware that it's expensive. Find yourself a good cosmetic surgeon with whom you have an excellent personal rapport. Don't be afraid to shop around to find the surgeon of your choice. Here are some things that may help you:

• Get a good recommendation. The best recommendation will be one from your own doctor, who may be able to give you an objective, professional opinion. Almost as good is a recommendation from a friend who has had cosmetic surgery, especially if you knew her before and afterward.

• Be careful when following up an advertisement from a newspaper or a magazine; contact your local or state medical society to find out whether the doctor is in good standing and is licensed to perform cosmetic surgery.

• A good surgeon will advise you on which operation will bring about the best results for you. Be suspicious of a surgeon who agrees to perform exactly the operation that you request without giving a professional opinion as to what you actually need.

• No good surgeon will give you a 100 percent guarantee of success. Some time should be taken to explain to you in detail exactly what the operation involves and what will hopefully be achieved, and to give a realistic estimate of the chances of success. Be skeptical about a surgeon who is not realistic about the results of the operation.

• Only entrust yourself to a surgeon with whom you strike up a good relationship from the very beginning. If you don't like the surgeon at your first visit, you're unlikely to later on.

• Your surgeon should answer all your questions in detail and show you drawings, pictures, and examples of past work, especially "before and after" photographs. Make sure you see a range of photographs so that you can see good, moderate, and poor results for the operation you are interested in. Ask what exactly the operation entails and what the possible complications are, when you will go into the hospital, and what type of anesthetic you'll have.

• A good surgeon should always take several photographs of your breasts to study exactly how and where to make the correction. If this hasn't been done, ask to know why. If you are not satisfied with the answer, don't be afraid to shop around for another surgeon.

BEING PREPARED FOR COSMETIC SURGERY

Having cosmetic surgery is a two-way contract between you and your surgeon. While the surgeon owes you service of a high standard, you ought to have thought out your decision in some detail and have a realistic view of what the procedure and the results will be like. Here are a few points for you to bear in mind before going ahead with any form of cosmetic surgery:

• There are occasionally certain preconditions for some types of surgery. These may include being of a certain age, being as slim as possible, having already completed your family, accepting that you probably won't be able to breastfeed subsequently, and being prepared to lose nipple sensation.

• The results of the operation might not be as good as you expect, and in a very few cases may not be good at all, so make sure that you are prepared for the possibility that things may not work out exactly as you had planned. In addition, you must accept that there is a possibility of complications that could delay your recovery.

• Immediately after the operation you will feel sore, there may be bruising, your skin may be swollen, and there may be redness, discomfort, or even pain for several days or possibly weeks.

• You may be completely immobilized for a short period of time following the operation or have your activities restricted. If you're highly motivated to have the operation, however, you should be able to cope with these temporary setbacks, but you must be prepared in advance.

• All operations leave scars behind them, though a good cosmetic surgeon will be careful to hide them in natural skin lines. Occasionally, however, they are still visible, and even after a year or so you can expect to have a fine tracery of silver lines around the nipple and a line from the nipple to the underpart of the breast. If you have any concerns whatsoever about scarring, you should talk in some detail to your surgeon about the chances of there being any after the breast surgery, and how extensive it will be.

All surgery carries some risk: you may react badly to the general anesthetic, develop a subsequent chest infection, and very, very rarely not survive the procedure. Be under no illusions – you are having a serious surgical procedure that, except in a very few instances, is entirely unnecessary. It could be argued that older women, whose hearts and chests are less fit and healthy than those of young women, run greater risks with surgery and anesthesia. Older women would also be well advised to have a mammogram before undergoing any form of plastic surgery, because of the increase in cancer risk with age.

TYPES OF SURGERY

There are several types of cosmetic surgery available for the breast. These include the correction of inverted nipples, breast-lift (mastopexy), breast enlargement (augmentation), and breast reduction.

Before agreeing to any of these major operations, make sure that you are fully aware of what the procedure will entail and the possible complications involved. Most important, you should be realistic about the probable outcome of the operation. Although it will change your appearance, it will not necessarily change your life.

INVERTED NIPPLES

Inverted nipples are so common that they can be thought of as a variation of normal (see p.44). In many cases, such nipples can be everted simply by the wearing of breast shells over a period of a few weeks (see p.45). If your breasts do not respond to the wearing of nipple shells, it could be that the nipple is being tethered down by a strap of fine tissue, which is nearly always caused by congenitally short ducts. If this is so in your case, you may find that surgery is the most helpful solution.

It's important for all women to be aware that this corrective procedure exists, but particularly so for teenagers, who can be painfully embarrassed by inverted nipples and for whom correction is very rewarding psychologically. Anyone considering this operation, however, should be aware that surgical intervention could make breastfeeding somewhat more difficult than normal, and if the ducts are cut, breastfeeding is impossible.

The operation Correction of an inverted nipple can easily be done under local anesthetic and requires only a few hours in the hospital. During the operation the surgeon pulls the nipple out from the breast and, while it is under tension, simply makes an incision around the nipple and into the tissue that is holding the nipple down. Cutting this tissue will allow the nipple to protrude. The procedure is a relatively simple surgical operation.

After-effects and follow-up You will be able to return to work two or three days after the operation, and your stitches will be taken out about two weeks later. You won't know for sure whether you can breastfeed until your breasts become active during pregnancy. There may be some loss of sensation in the breast and there is also a chance that the inversion will recur, but if this happens the operation can be repeated.

ASYMMETRY

No two breasts are the same, not even on the same woman, so all of us are asymmetrical to one degree or another. Some women, however, have very noticeable asymmetry of their breasts, which makes it difficult to find clothes that fit. Buying a decent bra may be difficult, too, especially if the breasts are

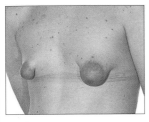

Before

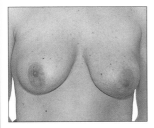

After

Asymmetry
It is quite normal for one breast to be slightly bigger than the other, but if the difference is very marked and distresses you, plastic surgery can give a more balanced appearance.

of different cup sizes. For women with a pronounced asymmetry of this kind, plastic surgery may be worthwhile, and there are three options: you can have the smaller breast augmented, the larger breast made smaller, or even a combination of the two. If the choice between augmentation and reduction is not a clear-cut one for you, read as much as you can about both operations. You may feel that you would rather not have an implant in your body; on the other hand, you may prefer augmentation to reduction, since it is less likely to involve a general anesthetic, and the scarring is significantly reduced.

Whatever operation you choose, bear in mind that an exact match after surgery is unlikely. An implant may stretch the nipple and areola, making those on the augmented breast noticeably larger than those on the other. Also, if you had a difference in nipple and areola sizes prior to the operation, this may still be the situation after surgery. As you grow older, the breast with the implant is likely to sag differently from the other breast. Given that any major differences in size and shape of your breasts have been corrected, however, these small discrepancies are unlikely to be all that noticeable to you or cause you any distress.

MASTOPEXY (BREAST-LIFT)

A breast-lift operation involves removing excess skin and raising the nipple. It can be combined with augmentation if your breasts are small or reduction if your breasts are very large. Without reduction, mastopexy is not very effective on large breasts, because gravity will pull them down.

Your expectations of the operation should be realistic. Mastopexy will not give you the pert breasts of a teenager, and in addition, the operation will leave scars. Discuss the operation in detail with your surgeon before you proceed. As with all breast operations, make sure you see "before and after" photographs of patients and ask to see a range of photographs so that you can check good, moderate, and poor results.

Ask for a description of the kind of cuts that are going to be made, and even get the surgeon to draw on your breasts where the scars will result. Your surgeon is not entirely in control of how the scars will look, because scars on some women are more prominent than on others. Make sure that you discuss fully with your doctor any possible complications that may arise both during and after the operation.

You should also bear in mind that your breast-lift, just like a face-lift, is by no means permanent; your breasts will continue to age and will eventually sag. Ask your surgeon if the technique to be used will give you the option of breastfeeding if this is important to you. It is advisable for you to have a mammogram before you go ahead with any type of surgery.

The operation Mastopexy can be carried out under either a local or general anesthetic, though a general anesthetic is more usual. The surgeon will need to remove excess skin and fat and move the nipple up. The operation will probably last in the region of two to two and a half hours.

After-effects and follow-up Mastopexy is usually very successful, and there are few side effects, though you may notice loss of sensation in your nipple and areola, and there is every chance that you will be able to breastfeed after the operation, unless the ducts are cut.

You can expect to have all the stitches removed after two weeks, and if you're an active person, you'll have full movement of your arms and shoulders and be able to resume sports after about three weeks. Although it may be slightly uncomfortable, it's advisable to wear a bra after the operation to support the inflamed breast tissues and skin and aid the healing process. You should be prepared to wear your bra day and night for at least three months after surgery. Your doctor will probably want to see you only after three months to make sure that no complications have arisen, but in most cases follow-up will not be necessary, providing the operation has achieved a satisfactory result.

MASTOPEXY

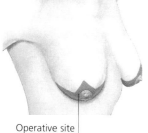

Operative site is marked out

1 The first step of a breast-lift operation is to mark the area of skin that is to be removed.

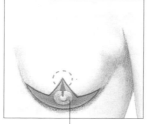

The areola is lifted up

2 Excess skin and fat is removed from the breast, and the nipple is raised to its new position.

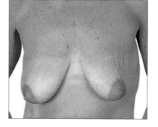

Before

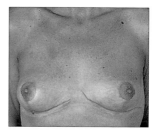

After

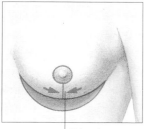

Skin edges are pulled together

3 The nipple is placed in its new position and the skin edges are pulled together and sewn.

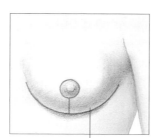

The skin is stitched together

4 Excess skin is removed from beneath the breast. The skin is then stitched together.

SCARS

After the operation you can expect to be left with some scarring around the areolae and under the breasts. Some techniques do not require an incision under the breasts, however (known as "vertical-scar mastopexy").

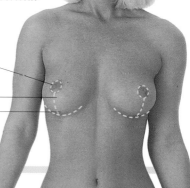

Around areola

From areola to base of breast

Underneath breast

BREAST REDUCTION

A sense of proportion is needed when you're deciding what size you would like your breasts to be, and your surgeon will have a good idea about what sizes are possible. The majority of women who want breast reduction opt for a size B, but it is not always easy to achieve an accurate result. There are two groups of women who look for breast reduction. The first group dislike their large breasts because of the inconvenience and the social embarrassment. The second group want cosmetic breast reduction to achieve well-positioned, firm breasts and are happy with a C or D cup as long as the breasts look good.

The operation While different surgeons have slightly different techniques for reducing the size of breasts, the basic operation is very much the same no matter who does the operation. It requires a general anesthetic, and it will probably take as long as four hours. Ask whether your surgeon is going to transpose your nipples or remove them and then graft them back.

The most commonly used method is the "keyhole" technique. The area of skin to be removed resembles the shape of a keyhole. If you wish to know exactly what's going to be removed, ask your surgeon to draw the shape on

REDUCTION

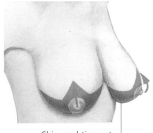

Skin and tissue to be removed

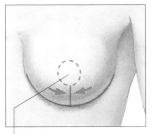

Nipple and areola under skin

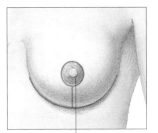

Nipple and areola in new position

SCARS
After the operation you can expect some scarring around the areolae, in a vertical line descending from the areolae and along the base of the breasts.

1 Tissue is removed from the base and sides of the breast, and the nipple and areola are moved up on a pedicle.

2 The skin edges are stitched together, leaving the nipple and areola temporarily inside.

3 A new nipple position is marked. The nipple is retrieved and stitched into its new position.

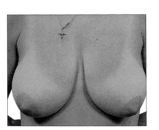

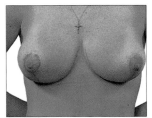

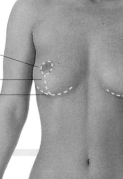

Around areola

From areola to base of breast

Underneath breast

Before

After

your breasts with a pen. You can also request that your nipple be preserved on a stalk of tissue – called a pedicle – and the tissue to be removed taken from the sides and the underside of this stalk. The nipple can then be lifted up and stitched into the breast at a higher level, and the flaps of skin underneath can be sutured together, resulting in reduction and some uplift. You will be left with scars surrounding the areola, in a line from the nipple to the underside of the breast and in the skin fold where the breast joins the skin of the chest.

After-effects and follow-up If the nipples are removed and grafted back on, then the sensation in your nipple and areola will certainly be reduced, as will your chances of breastfeeding. If, however, the nipple is lifted on a pedicle, you will have a small chance of still being able to breastfeed a baby.

This is a substantial operation, and you can expect to have some discomfort for several days following it. By the time you go home two or three days later, however, the pain should have largely subsided. Wear a bra day and night for support and to aid healing. The stitches should be removed within about two weeks, after which you could restart work. After a month you will be virtually back to normal. The results of the operation are usually extremely good.

Women who are motivated to have breast reduction surgery because of uncomfortable, pendulous breasts are nearly always more pleased with the results than those who are going for a purely cosmetic change.

Side effects are rare, but they do occasionally occur and include infection, which is possible with any operation. If the breasts are extremely large, the pedicle may carry an insufficient blood supply to keep the nipple and areola healthy, though this is extremely rare. Sensation in the nipple and areola may be reduced. There is no way that your surgeon can predict whether you will suffer loss of sensation after the operation, because your response to surgery is entirely individual. Even though your breasts have been reduced, if you gain weight, fat will be deposited and your breast size could increase again.

BREAST AUGMENTATION

Enlargement of the breasts is always accomplished with the aid of implants, which are inserted in front of or behind the muscles of the chest wall under the actual breast tissue. Implants have received a lot of media attention in recent years, and their safety has been questioned because of contracture (see p.114) and supposed links with autoimmune disorders. If you are considering breast augmentation, you owe it to yourself to become informed about these issues. I have outlined the current thinking on p.113, but your surgeon should be able to answer any questions you have.

The operation Augmentation surgery will take a minimum of 1½ hours, the length of the operation being largely determined by where the implant is placed. If it goes underneath the muscles of the chest wall, the operation will take less time than if it is placed underneath the breast tissue on the top of the muscle layer, because there is less bleeding in the former operation. You might want to stay in the hospital for 24 hours to recover from the anesthetic, but then you can go home. Usually you will be asked to return to the hospital within about ten days to have any stitches removed.

After-effects and follow-up Make arrangements to be off work for at least ten days or two weeks. Don't attempt to drive a car for a full seven days, and avoid overhead lifting for about four weeks. You should be back to normal in about three weeks, but it is best to avoid sports for about six weeks. You may feel more sensation than normal when touched, your nipples may feel numb, your breasts may feel uneven, and hot and cold sensations will feel a bit odd.

YOUR CHECKLIST BEFORE UNDERGOING BREAST AUGMENTATION

Breast augmentation is not a straightforward operation unattended by complications. You should therefore read as much as you can about it and talk to as many people as possible so that you go into it with your eyes open about what can go wrong. Have a detailed discussion as to what size you would like your breasts to be. Be realistic, though – if your frame is small and you already have tiny breasts, think twice before going for a D cup. Your surgeon will probably advise against it. The best prostheses now available are shaped and are of standard width. You will be measured for the appropriate size and shape

AUGMENTATION

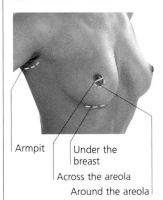

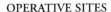

Armpit

Under the breast

Across the areola

Around the areola

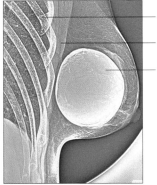

Ribs

Pectoral muscle

Implant

IMPLANTS
The round, white shape shown in the mammogram X-ray on the left is a silicone implant placed under the glandular tissue of the breast.

OPERATIVE SITES
The incision for an augmentation operation may be made in the armpit, around or across the areola, or under the breast. Scarring may occur in any of these areas, depending on which incision your surgeon uses.

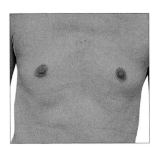

Before

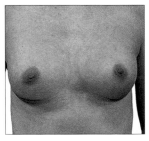

After

of these biodimensional prostheses. Make sure that your doctor checks for cysts in the breast that might require treatment in the future. It's difficult for a surgeon to interfere with the breast once an implant is in place. Discuss with your surgeon the possibility of contracture (see p.114) and ask where the scars will occur. Ask too if the incisions will interfere with future breastfeeding or sensation in the nipple and the areola, although the latter should affect only about 2 women in 100. Make sure that your surgeon tells you the size and the manufacturer of your implant, in case it needs replacing at a later date.

IMPLANTS

There are two types of implants available: fixed-volume implants and tissue expanders, where implant volume can be altered. Both types have a textured silicone shell filled with either saline (salt in solution) or silicone gel.

Fixed-volume implants are most commonly used for purely cosmetic surgery. Expanders are used in women who have had a mastectomy to allow the skin and tissue to stretch to accommodate the implant (see pp.190–91). The filling is injected through the skin into a valve attached to the implant, and the volume is increased gradually over several weeks. Once the breast has been expanded to the desired size and shape, the implant can be left permanently in position or replaced with a fixed-volume implant.

Saline or silicone? The likelihood of contracture is about the same with saline-filled implants, but there is no risk of silicone leakage. They don't, however, have the natural feel of silicone gel-filled implants. If leakage does occur in silicone implants, they will deflate and will need to be replaced. All implants used to be smooth on the outside, but these days a textured surface is preferred, as this seems to reduce the occurrence of contracture (see p.114).

New implant fillings Alternative implant-fill materials are currently being researched. It is hoped that these new materials will be capable of absorption by the body if leakage occurs, won't obscure mammography X-rays, and won't react with breast tissue. Types of materials being researched include gel-like solutions of water, salts, and organic polymers. One new implant, already available in some places, contains triglyceride, which is similar to body fat, and has a built-in electronic chip uniquely coded to identify the implant.

Breast cancer The link between silicone implants and cancer, which was suggested by the finding that silicone injected directly into rats will cause cancer, is entirely unproven. It's important to realize that we no longer inject silicone directly into breast tissue as we used to, and that data obtained from studies on rats can't simply be applied to human beings. Bear in mind, too, that implants have been around for over 30 years and have been used in nearly two million women, not to mention the large number of people who use other silicone products, such as contact lenses. The Food and Drug Administration (FDA) in the U.S. concluded in 1989 that "a carcinogenic effect in humans could not be completely ruled out, but if such an effect did exist, the risk would be very low." Breast surgeons around the world have found this statement reassuring enough to continue using silicone implants.

Autoimmune disease Silicone gel has been known to bleed out of the implant shell, and there have been sporadic reports of this causing connective tissue disorders like rheumatoid arthritis and systemic lupus erythematosus (SLE). These are tissue injuries resulting from autoimmune disorders, in which the body seems to become allergic to itself. A 1994 study from the Mayo Clinic in Rochester, Minnesota, doesn't rule out the link between connective tissue disorders and silicone implants, but it does show that the risk is very low. Nevertheless, in November 1994, the FDA banned the use of silicone implants, though the *New England Journal of Medicine*, one of the foremost and most influential in the world, felt that this was not medically justifiable. A more recent study, also reported in the *NEJM*, was carried out by doctors at Harvard University. Over the last 14 years they have found that connective tissue disorders are equally likely to occur in women who have not had implants and those who have. The American ban on silicone has not yet been lifted, although the implants are still used throughout the rest of the world.

Mammography Implants can make it difficult to read mammograms precisely (see p.64). Women who have a strong family history of breast cancer should probably avoid breast augmentation. It's a good idea for all women to have a mammogram before any plastic surgery is done. To get a good mammogram of a breast with implants the implant may have to be pushed aside, and the radiologist will need to take more than a single view.

CAPSULAR CONTRACTURE

The capsule of scar tissue that forms around an implant can be quite thin and pliable, but it may contract and become as hard as wood. One research study puts the possibility of some degree of contracture as high as 7 out of 10 at two to four years after surgery. Massaging the breasts may reduce the firmness, but if they are very hard, treatment can be quite complicated. Your surgeon can ease the tension by cutting a wider space around the implant, or if the implant is above the muscles of the chest wall, it can be removed and a new one inserted below the muscle, where contracture is less likely.

Other complications Breast pain, loss of sensation in the breast, difficulty with breastfeeding, infection, and movement and leakage of an implant are all known complications. A more uncommon one is rupture of the implant, which can occur spontaneously or through physical force such as a blow. You will need immediate surgery to remove all traces of silicone. Some authorities say half of all breast-augmentation patients will have some side effect by ten years after the operation; others estimate a one-in-three chance. None of these side effects, however, is life threatening.

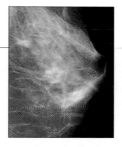

CHAPTER SEVEN

BENIGN BREAST CHANGES

Many changes in the breast reflect normal, harmless conditions. They do not necessarily indicate cancer or even disease. A woman should be helped to maintain a calm and rational response to benign breast changes, and to understand that the changes are the normal effects of her age, menstrual cycle, and lifestyle.

CHANGE OR DISEASE?

Cysts, solid lumps, and nipple discharge are all normal, harmless conditions that arise in the breast. Since there is no abnormality present, it's misleading to call such conditions "diseases," and well-informed doctors now use the term *benign breast change*. This is crucial to a woman for whom the word *disease* implies something abnormal or, worse still, dangerous. It's imperative that doctors too stop thinking of these conditions as disease because they have been trained to believe that disease justifies intervention. If your doctor refers to a breast condition in ambiguous terms, always ask for clarification of the terminology being used; if you don't understand what is being said, defer treatment until you receive a second opinion.

CLASSIFICATION

Until about 15 years ago breast conditions were not well understood, and there was confusion as to what was normal and what was abnormal. To confound both patient and doctor, conditions were inconsistently labeled, with the same labels being used to mean different things. The confusion was made worse when the terms *fibrocystic disease*, *fibroadenosis*, and *chronic mastitis* came to be used to describe the whole range of benign breast conditions.

As the spectrum of benign breast conditions contains one or two that are precancerous, the label *fibrocystic disease* was eventually applied to them, too. It was then only a matter of time before totally benign conditions were seen as precancerous. This led to misinterpretation in the media and great anxiety for women. Worst of all, however, doctors performed surgical operations on lumps that could have been left safely undisturbed. I believe that to prevent fear and confusion the terms *fibrocystic disease* and *fibroadenosis* should be abandoned; they have become so misused as to be meaningless, and have no place in the modern approach to breast conditions.

A NEW APPROACH

In Cardiff, Wales, in 1980, researchers developed a new and logical classification system for breast conditions that has a scientific basis. This system relates the most common breast conditions to normal changes that take place in the breast throughout a woman's lifetime and has been accepted in most countries where breast research takes place, including the US and the UK. It provides a rational explanation for practically all benign breast conditions. The researchers decided to rename benign breast conditions as "aberrations (changes) of normal development and involution (shrinkage)," known by the acronym ANDI.

Age and breast changes
The development of elements in the breast, and hence the kinds of benign breast change that are likely to arise, are closely related to age. The chart below shows the phases of development: lobule development between the ages of 10 and 25; glandular change under the influence of menstrual hormones between the ages of about 13 and 45; and involution or shrinkage of the milk ducts from about 35 years onward.

Normal breast changes through life

WHY ANDI?

The ANDI classification is based on two facts about benign breast conditions. First, most conditions relate to the normal pattern of breast development with its stages of growth and shrinkage. Second, each condition fits into one of three main periods of our fertile lives (puberty to 25 years, 25 to 35 years, and 35 to 55 years), so certain symptoms are more common at certain ages.

One example is the development of a fibroadenoma (see p.129), a common lump in teenagers and women in their 20s. A fibroadenoma is simply a breast lobule of unusual size, shape, and consistency. Seen under a microscope the cells from a normal lobule and a fibroadenoma look identical.

Other normal structures of the breast cause lumps in exactly the same way. Between the ages of 35 and 40, for example, cysts arise from milk glands as the glandular elements of the breast break down, forming tiny lakes of fluid inside the breast tissue. When a woman is in her 50s, right at the end of the growth continuum, dilatation of the milk ducts to the nipple (ectasia, see p.132) can occur and may result in nipple discharge.

Any woman can get breast cancer but age does play a role if you discover a lump. Under age 35, the chances are overwhelmingly that you've found an enlarged breast lobule (fibroadenoma) that is benign and nothing to worry about. If you're between the ages of 35 and 55, the chances are that the lump is an innocent cyst. But if you're over 55, cancer must be a possibility, and your doctor will take immediate steps to make a firm diagnosis.

In the light of these observations we can now interpret most benign breast conditions as age-related variations on the normal; they are therefore better thought of as aberrations or natural mistakes, not diseases. Such aberrations for most women are symptomless, so they rarely prompt us to see a doctor. Only a few cause symptoms, and even fewer lead to disease. Most never get beyond the state of being simply a variation on normal development.

Although ANDI is becoming widely accepted as an understandable and non-frightening term for these aberrations, some doctors use the term *benign breast changes* (BBC) or *benign breast disorders* (BBD) instead.

VARIATIONS ON THE NORMAL

As a way of illustrating the thinking that produced the new classification, I have created a chart (see pp.118–19) that sets out the most common breast changes by age group. You will see that for each condition there are three stages: normal development, which occurs in all women; possible aberrations, which occur in many women; and disease, which occurs in only a few women.

It should be obvious from the chart that what is normal and what is termed a disorder are not that far apart in most cases and should not give rise to anxiety. It's the next step, however, that doctors are concerned about – the borderline between a disorder and something that could turn malignant.

Only in one disorder does this question become important – hyperplasia, when excess cells become heaped up to form additional layers and the cells themselves look abnormal under the microscope (see p.155). This can happen

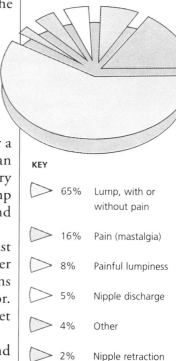

KEY

▷	65%	Lump, with or without pain
▷	16%	Pain (mastalgia)
▷	8%	Painful lumpiness
▷	5%	Nipple discharge
▷	4%	Other
▷	2%	Nipple retraction

Breast symptoms
The vast majority of benign breast disorders give rise to three main symptoms: a lump or lumpiness, pain, and nipple discharge. Taken singly, breast pain is the most common complaint being reported: at one breast clinic it appeared in 170 of 480 women (35 percent). Not all women who suffer breast pain ever seek help for it, however; it's thought that 7 out of 10 women suffer to some degree from pain, tenderness, and lumpiness.

in a lobule, duct, or cyst. In most instances there is still no increased risk of ever developing cancer, but in a few there is, and the risk depends on how abnormal the cells look. Even when cells become cancerous they may be what we call noninvasive, meaning they stay within the duct or gland and don't spread into the surrounding tissue. They will never kill you, so the diagnosis of cancer in this situation is never a disaster. A cancer of this kind is called an "in situ" cancer (see p.156).

ANDI AND DISEASE

There is no evidence that aberrations inevitably progress to disease. On the contrary, it seems that for this to happen some additional factor is needed – often an external one, such as smoking or an excessive alcohol intake. Duct ectasia (see p.132), for instance, rarely if ever develops into an infection or an abscess except where a woman smokes.

ANDI, therefore, usefully defines for us the spectrum from normal to minor aberrations, which encompasses most benign breast conditions brought about by minor physiological variations or even by chance. Disease, on the other hand, is associated with other possibly external influences that may trigger and promote the disease process. There are many such influences that have been identified as risk factors in breast cancer (see pp.143–50).

Breast change and life stages
Normal developmental changes in the breast can lead to harmless aberrations. These may in turn lead to benign conditions, but very rarely carry a risk of cancer.

TIME OF LIFE	NORMAL DEVELOPMENT	POSSIBLE ABERRATION (ANDI)
Early growth during fertile life, age 15–25	*Lobule formation*	*Enlarged lobule*
	Connective tissue formation	*Juvenile overgrowth*
Mature or midfertile life, age 25–40	*Hormonal effects on the breast of the menstrual cycle*	*Exaggeration of the ebb and flow of hormones each cycle*
Late or involutional part of fertile life, age 40 and over	*Dying back of lobules*	*Cysts*
	Scar formation inside breast	*Scars*
	Shrinkage of ducts behind the nipple	*Dilatation of duct with pooling of fluid, scarring around the duct*
	Increase in fat content	*Mild overgrowth of cells (hyperplasia, see p.155)*
		Atypical hyperplasia

YOUR CONCERNS

Almost all women fear breast cancer, so any breast symptom can cause alarm. Indeed, most women with breast symptoms seek reassurance even before they consider treatment. The women most at risk, and therefore those who should be most concerned about breast cancer, are those who are under 50 years old with a first-degree relative (mother or sister) who developed breast cancer at a young age or who developed cancer in both breasts (see p.146). As this is one area of cancer research that is likely to see great advances in the next few years, women in this category should always be treated at specialized breast centers, where thousands of cases are seen and doctors are very experienced. The women at greatest risk may be referred to special family-history breast centers for long-term assessment and follow-up to allay their fears. If you know you have a high risk of developing breast cancer, or are especially worried about your breasts, ask for referral to one of these centers; it's your right to do so. Should you develop cancer, don't accept treatment from a doctor who treats fewer than 30 breast cancers a year.

Women who are taking hormone replacement therapy are at no greater risk of developing breast cancer than are other postmenopausal women, and do not therefore need to have a routine follow-up at a breast center unless they or their doctor discover a lump.

WHAT YOU NOTICE	CONDITION THAT MAY DEVELOP	WILL ANDI TURN INTO INVASIVE CANCER?
Discrete lump	*Fibroadenoma, multiple fibroadenomas*	*No*
Excessive breast development	*None*	*No*
Pain and lumpiness of the breasts worst just before your periods. Lumps may be tiny and felt throughout the breast, or like separate small discrete lumps	*None*	*No*
A discrete lump	*None*	*No*
A hard ridge	*None*	*No*
Nipple discharge, nipple retraction	*Ectasia (see p.132), occasionally infection, rarely abscess formation*	*No*
Can't be seen or felt	*Unusual cellular overgrowth, rarely precancerous*	*Not necessarily*
Can't be seen or felt	*Can be precancerous*	*Possibly*

BREAST PAIN

Is breast pain real? To the 60 percent of women who experience mastalgia, to give it its medical name, the question seems ludicrous. Of course it's real – so real that for some women just having the breasts touched can be excruciating. Less than 20 years ago, however, breast pain, like gynecological pain such as menstrual cramps, was thought to be all in the mind; for decades it had been labeled neurotic, hysterical, and psychosomatic.

The unsympathetic and largely masculine trend of labeling breast pain as "a nervous disorder" was started by an eminent British surgeon, Astley Cooper, in the nineteenth century, but was still pervasive in the 1950s and 1960s. It was not until 1978 that Professor Robert Mansel of Cardiff, Wales, investigated this notion and reported that mastalgia sufferers were indeed psychologically stable and deserved a sympathetic approach to treatment. Largely due to Mansel's work, breast pain has become recognized as a legitimate complaint.

Types of breast pain Breast pain can be classified into two types: cyclical, which is associated with menstrual periods (see p.42), and noncyclical. Noncyclical pain may originate in the breast or in the nearby muscles and joints, in which case it is not true breast pain (see p.125).

HOW DOCTORS TREAT WOMEN WITH BREAST PAIN

Studies carried out in Manchester, England, indicate that women suffering from breast pain don't always get the understanding and treatment they deserve. It is clear that too many women seeking help are neither being examined or treated appropriately. Though over half the women studied had seen their family doctor, they still needed help and treatment. Other women avoided their doctor through fear or embarrassment. Still others had been met with the attitude that breast pain was a "nervous" or "neurotic" disorder.

Symptoms you should see a breast specialist about
Pain is not the only symptom that should make you visit a breast specialist. Any of these symptoms will require further investigation, and you should not be put off seeking the necessary help and advice.

PAIN	LUMP	NIPPLE DISCHARGE
Pain is associated with a breast lump	*You find a new, discrete lump*	*Discharge is associated with a lump*
Pain doesn't respond to your doctor's treatment	*You find a new lump in pre-existing general lumpiness*	*There is sufficient discharge to stain your clothes*
You are postmenopausal and have persistent pain in one breast	*A cyst persistently refills after being drained*	*You have bloodstained, persistent, or painful discharge*
	You notice asymmetrical lumpiness at the beginning of your menstrual cycle for more than one cycle	

It is still common for doctors to prescribe ineffective remedies for mastalgia – diuretics or even antibiotics. Some doctors suggest evening primrose oil in over-the-counter products, though the oil is believed to be effective only in high doses that are expensive unless obtained with a prescription.

EFFECTS ON LIFESTYLE

Although mastalgia can significantly disrupt daily life, even be incapacitating, not all women feel justified in consulting a doctor about it. In one study, 60 percent of women said they felt they had to cope without medical help. Although women may be reluctant to consult a doctor, the pain often causes them to call a breast helpline – indeed, mastalgia is the most common reason for calling such a helpline. Researchers from Europe have shown just how seriously breast pain can interfere with normal life. The figures below give the percentages of women who suffered from varying degrees of pain:

- sufficient pain to make them especially aware of the breasts   42%

- discomfort wearing a bra or light clothing   26%

- uncomfortable running up or down stairs   19%

- too uncomfortable for close physical contact   17%

- cannot bear any physical contact or pressure; pain would interrupt sleep and preclude sex   9%

FEAR AND BREAST PAIN

Even if breast pain does not interfere radically with normal life, fear of breast pain can be crippling because sufferers fear that cancer is the cause. Most women with mastalgia are much more worried about the possibility of cancer than about the pain itself. This includes the small number of women who suffer from incapacitating pain.

It's reasonable to be fearful of getting breast cancer, but it's not reasonable to be paranoid about it. If you have breast pain and are worried about it, you should visit your doctor. Bear in mind, though, that breast pain is rarely a symptom of breast cancer. And it would certainly be wrong to think that the worse the pain, the greater the chance that it's caused by malignancy. In fact, the opposite is true. The worse the pain, the less likely it is to be due to a malignant growth. Looked at this way, breast pain is a reassuring symptom, because its presence all but excludes breast cancer.

PSYCHOLOGY AND BREAST PAIN

All breast conditions can give rise to anxiety. For many women the symptoms are themselves stressful and as such may lead to psychological disorders. On the other hand, psychological disorders may show

Locations of pain
Pain that seems to be in the breast may in fact originate from some other part of the body, typically the bones or muscles. Locating the pain precisely helps a doctor decide whether the pain is true breast pain.

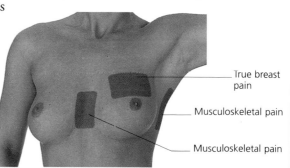

True breast pain

Musculoskeletal pain

Musculoskeletal pain

Breast pain Often made worse by stress, breast pain can also increase stress because of fear of cancer

Psychological stress Stress related to personality or a psychological disorder can make breast pain worse

Personality Stress can adversely affect personality, and some personalities are more sensitive to stress

Psychological disorder A psychological disorder can be worsened by the stress arising from breast pain

Cause and effect
Because mastalgia was once thought to have a psychosomatic origin, many studies have been done to investigate the relationship between breast symptoms, personality, and anxiety. Far from demonstrating that women who suffer breast pain are neurotic, such studies have demonstrated a complex relationship between breast symptoms and psychological problems, which can sometimes make it difficult to distinguish cause from effect.

up as, or be the cause of, breast symptoms, though in saying this I am not suggesting for a moment that the symptoms are imaginary.

Ironically, the highest levels of anxiety are found in women who are subsequently diagnosed as having purely benign disorders. Studies using internationally accepted methods for measuring anxiety also came up with the startling finding that the degree of stress felt by women with severe mastalgia is similar to that felt by women with operable breast cancer on the morning of surgery.

Given this degree of pain and anxiety, it is very important for women to realize that they can receive simple and effective treatment for mastalgia.

LUMPINESS AND BREAST PAIN

It used to be thought that lumpiness in the breasts, including cyclical lumpiness (see p.42), could cause breast pain and that, conversely, breast pain would eventually lead to lumpiness. Neither of these concepts has any medical foundation. When mammography was used to measure lumpiness, it was found that women with severe lumpiness had no more breast pain than women with no lumpiness at all. Then again, when women with mastalgia had ultrasound examinations, only half had lumpy breasts. Nor does the degree of lumpiness reflect the degree of pain that a woman experiences. Both lumpiness and pain are common, however, so it is hardly surprising that they frequently occur together. The association between pain and lumpiness is mainly true of cyclical pain.

As well as lumpiness, breast pain is commonly associated with swelling, hardening, and a feeling of tension in the breast. Your doctor may refer to this as engorgement, but it's not the same as the engorgement that a breastfeeding mother experiences when her breasts become overfull with milk.

CYCLICAL BREAST PAIN

The most common kind of breast pain is associated with the menstrual cycle and is nearly always related to hormones (see p.42). Pain is probably related to the sensitivity of breast tissue to hormones, and this can differ within a breast and between your two breasts. Hormones aren't the whole story, however, because in the majority of women the pain is more severe in one breast than in the other. Most women experience some degree of breast pain when their breasts become sensitive just prior to menstruation. Some women, however, may experience soreness and tenderness starting in the middle of the cycle with ovulation and continuing for about two weeks until menstruation takes place. Others find that this premenstrual soreness becomes even worse after the birth of their first child.

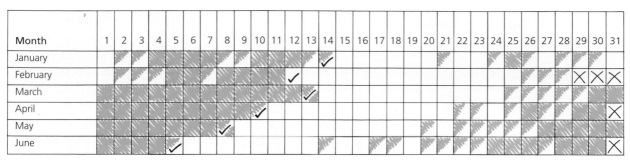

Month	1	2	3	4	5	6	7	8	9	10	11	12	13	14	15	16	17	18	19	20	21	22	23	24	25	26	27	28	29	30	31
January														✓																	
February												✓																	✗	✗	✗
March													✓																		
April										✓																					✗
May								✓																							
June					✓																										✗

 Severe pain   Mild pain   ✓ Period starts

The degree of pain varies. Sometimes it's hardly noticeable, but for some women the pain is so great that they wince when hugged, can't wear anything tight around their breasts, and can't lie on their stomachs. Sometimes the pain spreads out toward the armpit and occasionally down the arm to the elbow, which can cause women to fear that the pain is due to cancer or heart disease.

CAUSES OF CYCLICAL PAIN

There are many theories as to how hormones may be responsible for causing cyclical breast pain. One possibility is that the pain is due to changes in the production of prolactin, the milk-producing hormone, in response to changes in levels of thyroid hormone. We know that some women are very sensitive to thyroxine and respond to it by producing very high levels of prolactin, which induces breast pain. It's thought that abnormal "pulses" of prolactin may underlie cyclical mastalgia.

Breast pain can be affected by stress, and another theory suggests that it may be related to the many hormones that flood the body during stress. These include epinephrine, norepinephrine, hydrocortisone, and thyroid hormone.

French research has shown that mastalgia may occur when there's a lowered output of progesterone, thus changing the normal ratio of progesterone to estrogen in the second half of the menstrual cycle. Not all doctors agree with this theory, or with the practice of treating mastalgia with progesterone. At times in our lives when there are swings of hormones – puberty, pregnancy, or menopause – breast pain may be intense. During menopause this may be due to the ovaries secreting estrogen without producing progesterone; this changes the normal ratio of progesterone to estrogen.

TREATING CYCLICAL BREAST PAIN

If a man suffered breast pain 13 times a year he wouldn't hesitate to demand effective treatment. Neither should you. Every woman with mastalgia has the right to effective and safe relief from pain.

Evening primrose oil To be effective, evening primrose oil has to be taken in a large dose (3 grams daily). It also needs to be taken over a long period of time because its effect builds slowly – in most cases it takes as long as four months

Diagnosing cyclical pain
One of the first things your doctor will want to establish is whether the pain is cyclical or not. This chart, known as the standard Cardiff chart, allows you to record your pain each day – whether there is no pain, mild pain, or severe pain – so that you can see whether a pattern emerges. The first day of each menstrual period is marked with a tick. Put a cross through any dates that don't apply (such as February 29). After a couple of months, the relationship between the menstrual cycle and breast pain will emerge.

SEQUENCE OF TREATMENTS FOR CYCLICAL BREAST PAIN

INVESTIGATION	**NONCYCLICAL PAIN**
Doctor investigates pain using chart (see p.123)	Pain is treated according to cause (see p.126)
CYCLICAL PAIN	**MILD PAIN**
Decide whether any treatment is needed	If pain is mild, reassurance is often all that is required
SEVERE PAIN	**SUCCESSFUL**
Some doctors may try evening primrose oil first	Pain is cured – no further treatment is necessary
NO RESPONSE	**SUCCESSFUL**
If pain persists, doctor may go on to danazol	Pain is cured – no further treatment is necessary
NO RESPONSE	**SUCCESSFUL**
Bromocriptine may be tried if danazol is ineffective	Pain is cured – no further treatment is necessary
NO RESPONSE	**SUCCESSFUL**
If no response, possibly try tamoxifen or goserelin	Pain is cured – no further treatment is necessary

Sequence of treatments
The first step when you visit your doctor is to establish whether the pain really is cyclical. If it is, your doctor may prescribe evening primrose oil, moving on to other drugs only if there is no improvement after about four months. The arrows indicate the sequence of possible treatments.

to see if there is a good response to the treatment. It has very few side effects, which is why it is recommended. However, it can cause miscarriage and should not be taken by pregnant women.

Danazol With a success rate of nearly 80 percent, danazol is ideally the second line treatment. Despite this it is not suitable for everyone, as some women may experience side effects such as weight gain and irregular periods. Danazol is given in a dose of 200 milligrams daily for two months; if it has been effective after this time, the dose will be gradually reduced.

Bromocriptine Women who have not responded to treatment with evening primrose oil may go on to take bromocriptine. Bromocriptine works by blocking the hormone prolactin. It has about the same success rate as evening primrose oil, but it is more likely to have side effects (nausea, vomiting, and headache are among the most common). Giving it in a low dose at first – 1.25 milligrams nightly – and gradually increasing the dose to 2.5 milligrams twice daily can help to avoid these. You should always take bromocriptine with food.

NONCYCLICAL BREAST PAIN

There are two types of noncyclical breast pain: true breast pain, which comes from the breast but is unrelated to the menstrual cycle, and pain that is felt in the region of the breast but is actually coming from somewhere else. This latter kind nearly always involves the muscles, bones, or joints and for this reason is called musculoskeletal pain (see p.121). Two-thirds of noncyclical mastalgia is pain of musculoskeletal origin. Sometimes what appears to be breast pain is due to underlying lung or gall bladder disease.

DIAGNOSING NONCYCLICAL PAIN

Noncyclical breast pain is relatively uncommon and feels quite unlike cyclical breast pain. It doesn't vary with your menstrual cycle at all and is completely unrelated to hormones. It's nearly always confined to one spot, and you can usually point to exactly where the pain is – it's impossible to do this with cyclical breast pain. Recording your pain on a pain chart (see p.125) over a period of months will show that there is no cyclical pattern and that the pain is therefore unrelated to menstruation.

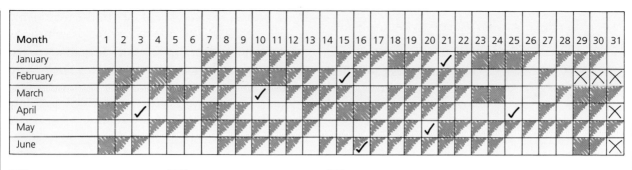

Month	1	2	3	4	5	6	7	8	9	10	11	12	13	14	15	16	17	18	19	20	21	22	23	24	25	26	27	28	29	30	31
January																					✓										
February															✓														✕	✕	✕
March										✓																					
April			✓																					✓							✕
May																			✓												
June															✓																✕

Severe pain Mild pain ✓ Period starts

If your doctor suspects noncyclical pain while examining you, you may be asked to lean forward so that the breast falls away from the chest. This helps to clarify whether the pain is located in the breast or in the chest wall. As with cyclical pain, a proper diagnosis is important; otherwise you may worry needlessly about breast cancer or your heart.

TRUE NONCYCLICAL BREAST PAIN

Some benign breast conditions may be associated with true breast pain. Burning or stabbing pains centred around or under the nipple are nearly always due to dilatation of the ducts (duct ectasia, see p.132) and tend to run an intermittent though harmless course.

A tender spot with occasional stabbing pain or an ache is common. Its cause is unknown, but it is no reason for anxiety. The pain can be relieved by an injection of local anaesthetic mixed with prednisone to help to reduce any inflammation. A cyst (see p.127) occasionally underlies a tender spot.

PAIN OF NONBREAST ORIGIN

Pain originating in the chest wall or spine may be felt in the breast area. The most usual cause is a form of arthritis, called costochondritis, which affects the ends of the ribs where they join the breastbone – a condition called Tietze's syndrome. If your pain is worse when you take a deep breath or press on your breastbone and ribs, it's probably this kind of arthritis. Taking an analgesic such as paracetamol or a nonsteroidal anti-inflammatory drug is often effective, which confirms the diagnosis.

Very occasionally, pain felt close to the breast originates from a pinched nerve in the neck. An X-ray of the cervical spine will reveal a condition called spondylosis, the natural erosion of the joints between the vertebrae due to aging. Another possibility is spondylitis, which means that there's some inflammation of the intervertebral joints.

In both of these conditions, spurs of new bone are laid down on the sides of the vertebrae and press on the nerves. The resulting pain may be felt in the neck, shoulder, chest, arm, or hand. Treatment includes analgesics to relieve the pain, manipulation and physiotherapy, and specific exercises designed to strengthen the muscles of the neck and shoulders.

Charting noncyclical pain
A pain chart makes it easy to identify noncyclical pain. No clear pattern emerges, and there is no relationship between the pain and the beginning of each menstrual period (marked with a tick). Put a cross through days that do not exist (February 29, for example).

Though rare, inflammation in the veins (phlebitis) of the breast, called Mondor's syndrome, causes pain much like that of an infection or an abscess. Careful examination may reveal the inflamed vein, which feels somewhat like a string under your fingertips. This condition is not harmful – a clot hardly ever escapes from an inflamed vein. Treated with hot and cold compresses and analgesics, it will subside in about a week.

SELF-HELP

Although I firmly believe that all women with mastalgia should receive medical treatment if they want it, there are self-help remedies that are worth trying. These remedies are in no way dangerous and are easy to implement.

Cyclical pain
• Vitamin E is said to help, though this is unproven.

• Water retention doesn't cause cyclical mastalgia, but it can make it seem worse if you're generally retaining fluid premenstrually. You might try taking naturally occurring diuretics such as parsley and capsicums. Coffee is one of the most powerful diuretics known and could greatly help to eliminate fluid.

• Early research suggests that a diet low in animal fat can reduce cyclical mastalgia. Although this is still unproven, such a diet is healthy anyway.

Treatments for noncyclical pain
The location and character of the pain offer important clues to the cause. In almost all cases, simple treatment measures will be successful.

Any breast pain
• Invest in a good support bra that is comfortable enough to wear at night.

• Some women find mental techniques such as deep relaxation, meditation, and visualization helpful. Hypnosis remains controversial, but with an expert practitioner results can be as good as with oil of evening primrose.

PAIN	CAUSE	TREATMENT	SUCCESS RATE
Around the breastbone	*Costochondritis, Tietze's syndrome*	*Analgesic, anti-inflammatory drug*	*Very good*
Localized pain in the side of the chest wall	*Tenderness of the pectoralis major muscle*	*Injection*	*Very good*
Diffuse pain in the side of the chest wall	*Viral infection with chest pains and fever*	*Nonsteroidal anti-inflammatory drug*	*Quite good*
Burning or stabbing pain round the nipple	*Duct ectasia (see p.132)*	*Analgesic*	*Good*
Tender spot in the breast with associated pain	*Unknown, occasionally associated with a cyst*	*Injection of anesthetic and prednisone, treatment of cyst (see p.131)*	*Good*
Drawing sensation round the outside of the breast	*Inflamed veins (Mondor's syndrome)*	*Compresses, analgesics*	*Good*

BREAST LUMPS

The most common breast lumps belong to a group of harmless conditions that have no sinister implications whatsoever but can cause anxiety if you don't understand how they arise and develop. Every woman has a lump (or general lumpiness) of one sort or another, though it may often be too small to feel. Practically all lumps are merely a variation of normal; they do not develop into cancers, and they won't kill you. There is no actual disease. This is very important information for all women, because on discovering a lump in their breasts they can be reassured that it probably belongs in the harmless category.

There are only two kinds of common benign breast lump: cysts and fibroadenomas. These lumps are not diseases – they're part of the normal changing growth pattern of the breasts throughout our lives (see p.116). There is a third type called a pseudolump which, as its name implies, isn't really a breast lump at all.

TRIPLE ASSESSMENT OF BREAST LUMPS

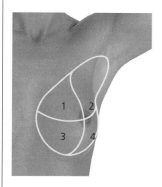

PHYSICAL EXAMINATION
Your doctor will palpate the breast and note the location of the lump (left). He or she will also examine the armpit for swollen lymph nodes.

1 Upper inner quadrant
2 Upper outer quadrant
3 Lower inner quadrant
4 Lower outer quadrant

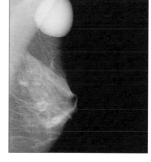

ULTRASOUND
Physical examination alone won't reveal whether the lump is solid or fluid-filled. An ultrasound scan will, however, make this distinction, and may pick up other lumps that are too small to feel. This ultrasound image (left) shows a large cyst.

FNAC
Fine-needle aspiration cytology (FNAC) is used to sample cells from the lump (right). Under mammographic guidance, or ultrasound if the lump can't be felt, a needle is inserted into the lump. If fluid is withdrawn, the lump is a cyst; the fluid can be aspirated and the lump will disappear. If the tumor is solid, the cells removed are spread on a glass slide (a smear) for staining and microscopic examination.

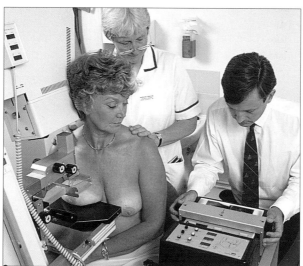

FNAC | Cells or fluid are withdrawn with a needle

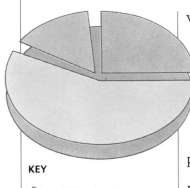

Minimum intervention
At a breast center where
women with solid breast
lumps were offered the
option of keeping their lump
intact if it turned out to be
benign, the results were as
shown above. Further
investigation or monitoring
was needed in 25 percent
of cases, and 75 percent were
definitely benign; altogether,
13 percent opted for surgery
and 62 percent decided to
keep their lumps.

We have no idea why these noncancerous lumps appear, although they're probably related in some way to variations in hormone production. Cysts and fibroadenomas grow only during a woman's fertile years, though they may be detected years later. They occur at the opposite ends of the hormonal spectrum, fibroadenomas being most common in the early part of a woman's fertile life and cysts during midfertile life.

A pseudolump can occur at any age and is nearly always extreme normal lumpiness, but it should be checked to make certain that all is well. (Other pseudolumps, such as the end of a rib or scar tissue, are discussed on p.62.)

LUMPINESS

A special word here about lumpy breasts. Lumpiness in both breasts is never sinister and needs no treatment, especially if it's worse premenstrually. Some doctors still dub it fibrocystic disease, which all experts agree is a misnomer. The danger is that some doctors still believe fibrocystic disease to be generally precancerous, whereas this is very rarely so. Once a doctor is thinking this way, however, preventive measures may be recommended – even bilateral mastectomy (complete removal of both breasts). If this is suggested to you, get a second opinion from a breast specialist. Bilateral mastectomy is hardly ever justified for lumpy breasts.

TRIPLE ASSESSMENT OF BREAST LUMPS

If you consult your family doctor with a breast lump, you will be referred to a breast specialist who will first try to establish whether the lump is benign or malignant by obtaining as much information about it as possible. To do this, doctors use a "triple assessment" approach: that is, using manual examination, mammography or ultrasound, and fine-needle aspiration cytology (see p.127) to check out the lump.

Because this approach is so thorough, false positives and false negatives are exceedingly rare. If cytology ever reveals malignant cells, your doctor will move on to biopsy (see p.160). Whether the cells are benign or malignant, surgeons will remove any lump in the breast of a postmenopausal woman.

RULING OUT CANCER

Breast cancer is rare in women under the age of 35, whatever the symptoms. If you're under 35, the odds are that your lump is a fibroadenoma regardless of size. If you find a new – and the emphasis is on *new* – discrete lump, your doctor will always refer you to a hospital for assessment. The presence of a lump overrides any other symptom, and you should expect your doctor to act accordingly, whether he or she believes the lump to be cancer or not. All doctors have the same priority – to exclude cancer.

The picture may be unclear if you already have some lumpiness in your breasts, because this occasionally obscures a very small cancer. If you're under 35 and if your other breast is also lumpy, cancer is unlikely – in fact, even if the lump is new, large, discrete, and mobile, cancer is most improbable. Between the ages of 35 and 55, the lump is probably a cyst – this can be confirmed immediately with FNAC (see p.127). Cysts are uncommon in women over 55, when the risks of developing cancer increase.

KEEPING THE LUMP

Excellent research done in Europe shows that the majority of women with benign breast disorders are happy to forego surgery once they have been reassured that the condition is indeed benign. This is sensible and humane, especially as there is no connection between malignant change and most benign breast conditions. As it is now possible to identify the vast majority of benign lumps without surgical removal, you have the right to keep your lump undisturbed. The only exception is a cyst where the simple procedure of FNAC will collapse and cure it. Most doctors will be happy to leave your lump untouched if the following are true:

- on examination, the lump feels smooth and is mobile

- mammography or ultrasound shows that the lump looks harmless

- FNAC shows nothing untoward

- follow-up examinations after three and six months show no change in the size or appearance of the lump; although some doctors do not require follow-up examinations, you should always return if you notice any changes.

FIBROADENOMAS

Common in teenagers and women in their 20s, fibroadenomas are simply overdeveloped lobules and are completely benign. You don't always need to have one removed, as long as you agree to a further ultrasound scan and examination in six months' time. The majority of women, when offered excision or observation, opt for the latter.

LOCATIONS OF FIBROADENOMAS

Although fibroadenomas can occur anywhere in the breast, they are often found near the nipple and are slightly more common in the left breast than in the right. No matter which breast they appear in, however, they are far more likely to occur in the upper outer quadrant and are seldom found in the lower ones.

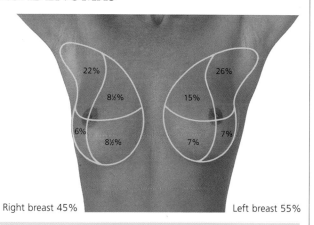

22%   26%

8½%   15%

6%

8½%   7%   7%

Right breast 45%   Left breast 55%

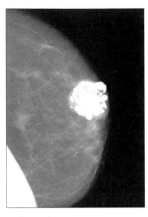

Fibroadenoma
This mammogram shows the well-defined outline of a fibroadenoma. Deposits of calcium around the lump account for its dense white color on the image.

Fibroadenomas can be very large – they vary from pea size to larger than a lemon. While they can grow anywhere in the breast, quite often they're found near the nipple. They feel smooth and firm and quite distinct, and move freely in your breast. Most doctors can recognize one simply by feeling it, but the diagnosis should be clinched with mammography or ultrasound and fine-needle aspiration cytology (FNAC).

Although they are most common in young women, fibroadenomas can occur at any age up to menopause (or later if you are on HRT). Most women who get a fibroadenoma will never get another one, but a few women will have several over their lifetime. It is also possible to have more than one at a time or a single large fibroadenoma involving more than one lobule. In very rare cases there may be a tendency for them to run in families.

TREATMENT

Once the diagnosis is confirmed, you can decide whether or not you want to have the lump removed (see p.129). Most doctors in the past recommended removal of all fibroadenomas, irrespective of age and other considerations. Yet most fibroadenomas come to nothing and shrink, and many go undiscovered, so it's not unreasonable for your doctor to take a flexible attitude according to your age. If you're not worried, there's no need to have it removed. Where there is no clear result from cytology or ultrasound, however, removal is wise for all lumps. If you're under 25, cancer is so rare that a typical fibroadenoma can be left without risk, but you can have it removed if you wish. Opting to avoid surgery will mean your doctor will need to see you again in six months to monitor the lump. Fibroadenomas usually remain static, but if yours enlarges you can have it removed at any time. Young women are often advised to watch and wait rather than undergo surgery and the resulting scarring.

Surgery, when it's done, is very simple and is usually conducted under local anesthetic. The surgeon will make a small incision over the lump and remove it. The incision will be made along the natural tension lines of the skin, and the scars should be virtually invisible when they heal.

Surgical removal of a very large fibroadenoma, however, can leave the breast misshapen. If you're having one removed, first discuss with your specialist the possibility of having your breast surgically refashioned, either at the time of the operation or later. This option will be available in most breast centers. If not, the fibroadenoma can be removed through an incision in the skin fold under the breast to give the best cosmetic result.

FIBROADENOMAS AND CANCER

Extremely large fibroadenomas – those larger than a lemon – may undergo cancerous change at their centers. This kind of cancer grows slowly, does not spread to other parts of the body, and does not kill. The fact that some large fibroadenomas may become cancerous is therefore not a justification for removing all fibroadenomas, especially as this kind of change is rare. Having a fibroadenoma does not in itself increase your risk of developing cancer.

CYSTS

The blockage of glands as they change through life causes cysts, so they're a variation of normal breast anatomy, not a disease. A cyst is a fluid-filled sac similar to a large blister buried in breast tissue. When you feel it you can usually detect its smooth outline, and you may even be able to bounce it between two fingers as you push the fluid from side to side. This is particularly so when the cyst is near the surface; when it's buried deep in breast tissue, however, it will simply feel like a hard lump.

Quite often a cyst will seem to appear suddenly – even overnight. This is a very reassuring sign, because anything that appears so suddenly is almost certainly harmless. Cysts are most commonly found in women in their 30s, 40s, and 50s with the peak just prior to the menopause. It's possible, though rare, for cysts to occur in young women or in postmenopausal women.

Your doctor may be able to identify a lump as a cyst simply on physical examination, but most breast specialists will wish to confirm the diagnosis by following up with a mammogram or an ultrasound examination. Your doctor will then probably suggest fine-needle aspiration cytology (FNAC, see p.127) as the next step to confirm the diagnosis.

TREATMENT

With cysts, FNAC serves as both diagnosis and treatment. Aspiration can be done quickly, simply, and painlessly as a routine procedure in the breast clinic. No local anaesthetic is necessary, as all you will feel is a needle prick. The needle is pushed through the skin into the cyst, which is then aspirated into a syringe and thus collapses and disappears. The whole procedure may be carried out under ultrasonic guidance, allowing you to watch as your doctor inserts the needle and aspirates the cyst and it disappears. Large cysts that are easily felt can be aspirated without the help of ultrasound.

The fluid from the cyst can be any color – brown, yellow, greenish, or milky white. (In breastfeeding women a milk-filled cyst can form; this is called a galactocele.) Studies have shown that there is no point in the aspirated fluid from the cyst being examined, because the risk of cancer is so minute. If the fluid is bloodstained, it is sent to the laboratory for analysis of the sediment.

CYSTS AND CANCER

Cysts are rarely malignant, or not harmfully so. In a very few cases, a small cancer may grow inside the cyst, but it usually doesn't spread beyond the cyst into the surrounding breast tissue, and it cannot kill you. Nevertheless, your doctor will operate on the cyst and remove it completely if there is any evidence of cell growth found in it. If you have a simple cyst, you will not have any increased cancer risk.

Occasionally cysts reform. If this happens, you should return to your doctor to have the cyst aspirated; although the cyst is harmless in itself, it could obscure other changes in the breasts. A cyst that persistently refills after being drained carries a slightly increased risk of cancer.

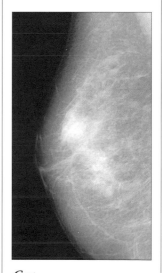

Cyst
Mammography will detect a cyst, but cannot distinguish between it and other breast lumps. Here the cyst appears as an irregular white area behind the nipple.

NIPPLE CONDITIONS

Benign disorders affecting the nipple are less common than lumpiness and pain, but can be equally worrying; like all breast complaints they warrant prompt diagnosis to eliminate a rare cancer and decide appropriate treatment.

DILATATION OF THE MILK DUCTS – ECTASIA

Just as normal changes in the breast lobules can result in the formation of fibroadenomas in young women, and changes in glands lead to cysts later in life, so the normal involution of milk ducts in a woman's 40s and 50s can lead to nipple disorders. The underlying change in the normal anatomy of ducts as a woman grows older is ectasia, or dilatation. Frequently this leads to blockage of the ducts with pooling of fluid behind the blockage. Infection may lead to chronic inflammation, and sometimes an abscess forms.

Ectasia of the milk ducts is a phenomenon that occurs in the last part of the development cycle in the breast – involution or shrinkage. This condition is normal and so may affect both breasts, but it should not normally cause any change in the nipple. If an infection develops and affects the dilated ducts, surrounding inflammation (periductal mastitis) can lead to the formation of scar tissue that contracts and draws the nipple in (inversion).

Ectasia is normal, but an infection that arises from it is not. Fortunately, as a complication of ectasia it hardly ever occurs except in women who smoke, and it won't heal if a woman continues to smoke. We don't understand the reason, but the connection is clear. Nipple infection is therefore another good reason to give up cigarettes.

PROBLEMS ARISING FROM DUCT ECTASIA

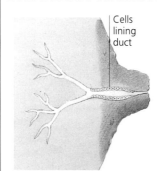
Cells lining duct

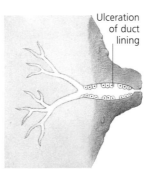
Ulceration of duct lining

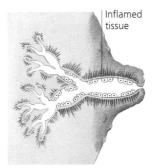
Inflamed tissue

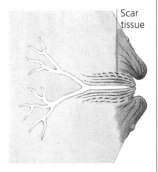
Scar tissue

1 **NORMAL ECTASIA** *As the breasts age, the ducts behind the nipple become dilated, leading to stagnation of fluid inside them.*

2 **DISCHARGE** *Stagnating fluid inside the duct causes the lining to become ulcerated. There may be bloodstained discharge from the nipple.*

3 **INFLAMMATION** *Fluid leaks through the damaged duct lining into the surrounding tissue, causing painful inflammation.*

4 **INVERTED NIPPLE** *The tissue behind the nipple becomes scarred and shrinks, pulling the nipple in.*

These two factors – the normal dilatation of the ducts with aging, and inflammation or infection of the ducts – account for most nipple problems in women over 50, including recurrent subareolar abscesses (infected lumps) and nipple retraction. Occasionally ectasia causes breast pain.

INFLAMMATION

Infection is the usual cause of inflammation around the ducts (periductal mastitis), but inflammation can also occur without infection; this form is thought to be due to irritation by stagnant secretions leaking from a dilated duct. A bacterial infection may result in chronic inflammation, and may cause the tissue behind the nipple to stand out and be manifested as a lump – this is known as a granuloma. Such an infection can be difficult to root out, even with a course of antibiotics, so an abscess or a fistula (a seeping abscess with a permanent opening to the skin) may form. Whatever the cause of the mastitis, the end result is the same – gradual retraction of the nipple.

NIPPLE DISCHARGE

This third symptom of breast conditions is far less common than pain and lumps (see p.117). Bear in mind that nipple discharge that appears only if the breast and nipple are squeezed is of no consequence. It's also normal for women who have had children and have not yet entered menopause and for women who smoke to produce nipple secretions.

The risk of cancer in a woman with nipple discharge is very low, especially if both breasts are involved. In establishing the cause, it's important to find out whether the discharge is coming from one duct or several.

DIAGNOSIS

To evaluate nipple discharge, your doctor will perform a biopsy of the duct, removing tissue under the nipple as well. Mammography often reveals the characteristic coarse calcification of duct ectasia: little needle-shaped deposits of calcium around and pointing toward the nipple. Surgical removal of the involved ducts may be suggested if the discharge is embarrassing.

If a lump is found in conjunction with nipple discharge, investigation of the lump (see p.127) overrides any other consideration and takes priority. A lump beneath the areola in a breastfeeding woman is nearly always due to lactational mastitis (see p.134) complicated by an abscess.

MULTIPLE DUCT DISCHARGE

This is nearly always benign, being due to simple changes like ectasia. Discharge of this kind is best left alone unless, as rarely happens, it's profuse and sufficient to cause staining of clothes and embarrassment. Discharge caused by ectasia can be whitish, brown, gray, or green; it can also be watery or very thick. Surgical removal of the dilated or infected ducts will not be undertaken lightly; it can leave a woman unable to breastfeed and affect the sensation in the nipple and areola.

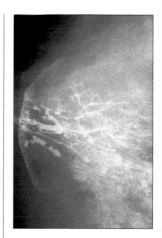

Dilatation of ducts
To produce this X-ray image, a contrast medium has been injected into the milk ducts so the pattern of dilatation shows up clearly.

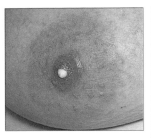

Milky discharge
The breasts can sometimes secrete milk in a woman who is not breastfeeding. This condition is called galactorrhea.

Occasionally, nipple discharge due to ectasia is accompanied by inflammation around the ducts, leaving the areolar skin red, hot, and hard. If left untreated, this can lead to fistulae, though mostly in heavy smokers.

SINGLE-DUCT DISCHARGE

To doctors, discharge coming from a single duct is more significant than from several ducts but, provided that mammography shows no abnormality, surgery will not be required. Bloodstained discharge is usually due to a small benign papilloma (a wartlike growth) growing inside a duct or an ulcerated duct. The affected duct can be surgically removed and will reveal a harmless cauliflowerlike structure. Very occasionally a bloody discharge will be due to a ductal cancer; this doesn't have serious implications, however, as this type of cancer is usually noninvasive (see p.156).

GALACTORRHEA

Milky discharge from both nipples, when it is not related to breastfeeding, is called galactorrhea. It is usually due to increased levels of the milk-producing hormone prolactin. Galactorrhea is often accompanied by amenorrhea (absence of menstrual periods) and can be caused by tranquilizers, marijuana, or very high doses of estrogen. Sometimes a small tumor of the pituitary gland in the brain (where prolactin is produced) is responsible, and this can be treated with bromocriptine (see p.124) or, rarely, surgical removal.

NIPPLE INFECTIONS

The milk ducts are vulnerable to infection because bacteria can enter from the outside. Although such infections are unpleasant and often painful, they can be treated and are almost never a sign of something more sinister.

LACTATIONAL MASTITIS

Nipple infections in a breastfeeding mother are the most common type. They nearly always arise from cracked, sore nipples; bacteria from a baby's mouth enter the lactiferous ducts through cracked skin and multiply rapidly in the milk. Occasionally, infection can result from a blocked duct. In either case, the breast becomes hard, hot, reddened, and painful.

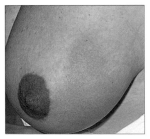

Mastitis
Most common in mothers who are breastfeeding, breast infections cause pain, inflammation, and a large, red, shiny patch on the skin.

Treatment Antibiotics combat the infection and analgesics deal with pain; neither should affect the baby. The breast should be rested for as short a time as possible because the baby's sucking keeps the milk flowing and helps to overcome the infection; milk should be expressed in the meantime to keep the supply going. About 1 infection in 10 goes on to form an abscess, which must be drained in the hospital, under general anesthetic if necessary. The wound is left open with a wick in place to facilitate draining, and a dry dressing is placed on top. Once the abscess has been drained and the pain has subsided, it's possible to breastfeed again. Sometimes ultrasound will show a small abscess, which can be treated by aspirating the pus through a needle.

Effects of smoking
The percentage of smokers with ectasia, a normal condition, is comparable to that in the population at large. Smokers, however, form the majority of women suffering from ectasia-related conditions: mastitis, abscesses, and fistulae.

KEY

Nonsmokers

Smokers

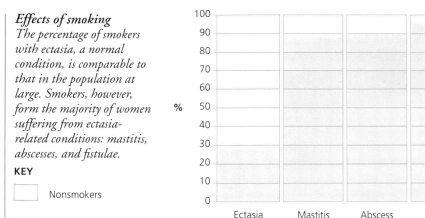

Ectasia and related complications

NONLACTATIONAL MASTITIS

Nipple infections are very rare in women who are not breastfeeding. Those most at risk are women whose immune systems are compromised, diabetics, and women who have had breast surgery.

CHRONIC SUBAREOLAR INFECTIONS

Long-term infections of the breast around the areola usually affect women in their early 30s, and are due to inflammation around the ducts. Smoking has been implicated as the most important cause, but it is not understood how smoking damages the ducts. Untreated, the area becomes inflamed, and an abscess may form. A mammary duct fistula is then a possibility if the abscess breaks down at the edge of the areola, and this can give rise to a permanent opening through the skin.

Treatment Antibiotics are the treatment of choice, but these infections are notoriously difficult to treat, especially if the patient continues to smoke. If the abscess fails to heal, an ultrasonic scan will determine its extent, and FNAC will exclude an underlying cancer. The abscess can be drained, but it may recur. A fistula must be surgically cut out.

If the abscess is very large, or the nipple has become badly inverted, or the infections recur even after removal of the fistula, larger-scale surgery may be recommended. Surgery may be disfiguring, so seek a second opinion – some doctors have been known to recommend mastectomy for recurrent abscesses! Most women are happy with major duct excision if they are forewarned of consequences such as lopsided breasts and loss of nipple sensation.

SKIN CONDITIONS

The skin of the breasts is thin and sensitive but, provided proper care is taken (see p.50), there is no reason why it should be more prone to problems than skin elsewhere. The nipple and areola, with their complex internal structure, glands, and duct openings, are the most prone to disorders.

CRACKED NIPPLES

During breastfeeding, the skin around the nipples is exposed to milk and vigorous sucking, both of which can damage the skin. Prevention is the best approach: the nipples should be gently dabbed clean after each feeding, and a baby who is latched on properly will not need to suck hard to feed well. Applying a drop of baby lotion to your breast pad can also help. If the nipples do become cracked, it is important to get advice on positioning the baby correctly on the breast and taking her off the breast gently – this is achieved by pushing down gently on the baby's chin to break the airtight seal between her mouth and the nipple. Treatment needs to be prompt, as cracked nipples are vulnerable to infections (see p.134).

ECZEMA

Scaly, red, itchy patches on the breast and nipple may be associated with generalized eczema elsewhere on the body, or can be localized entirely around the nipple and areola. Classically, eczema starts on the areolar skin and later spreads to the nipple. It usually appears on both nipples. It develops quite quickly and may clear up but then recur. The involved skin is usually moist, and the patch of eczema is likely to have an irregular outline. Eczema will normally respond to 1 percent hydrocortisone cream.

PAGET'S DISEASE

Although it looks like eczema, Paget's disease is actually a form of very slow-growing breast cancer. It tends to be associated with the in situ form of cancer (see p.156). Although it's not a benign condition, I mention it here because it's important to consider the possibility of Paget's disease whenever eczema of the nipple occurs. It can sometimes be distinguished from eczema just by looking: it invariably starts on the nipple as a nonscaly, moist, erosive patch with a florid raw red surface and definite outline and profuse discharge. It rarely affects both nipples.

Another distinguishing characteristic is that Paget's disease develops slowly and persistently – it won't clear up and then recur, like eczema. If Paget's disease is suspected, your doctor may recommend a biopsy and mammogram.

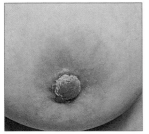

Paget's disease
A form of breast cancer that initially affects the nipple, Paget's disease shows up as itchy, scaly skin, and so is easily confused with eczema.

AREOLAR GLAND DISORDERS

The areolar skin contains three kinds of glands, and each can lead to problems. The apocrine sweat glands can become infected and form cysts; the sebaceous glands can form sebaceous cysts; and the accessory mammary glands can discharge or become infected.

TREATMENT

Infection of the sweat glands (hidradenitis suppurativa) can usually be cleared with an antibiotic cream, but the glands very often have to be removed if the infection persists. Cysts can be surgically removed under a local anesthetic if they are troublesome. Discharge and infection usually respond to antibiotics.

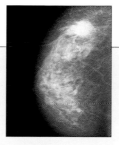

CHAPTER EIGHT

BREAST CANCER

Understanding the causes and effects of a disease such as cancer can greatly improve our chances of avoiding it altogether or defeating it should it occur. Knowledge of risk factors can help women make lifestyle changes to reduce their own risk. Modern techniques, such as grading and staging, mean that doctors can tailor treatment to the individual patient.

UNDERSTANDING BREAST CANCER

I have set myself several goals in writing about breast cancer. By far the most important message I want to communicate to you is that cancer of the breast need not be fatal. Only 1 breast lump in 10 ever turns out to be cancerous, and of those that do, a considerable number are of the noninvasive type – that is, they do not spread beyond their place of origin and therefore cannot kill. A cancer that is less than ½ inch (1 centimeter) in diameter – and this can be detected by self-examination or through routine mammographic screening – is still at a very early stage; there is therefore only a small chance that it has spread and less risk of its being fatal. One of the main aims of this chapter, therefore, is to curb the panic that may grip you when you discover a lump, so that you seek advice immediately and give yourself the best chance, rather than succumb to the paralyzing fear that the prospect of cancer may bring.

Another of my aims is to demystify cancer: I will explain what cancer is, describe how cancerous cells behave, how they differ from normal cells, and how environmental or internal triggers can prompt a normal cell to become cancerous. Of all the different types of cancer, breast cancer has probably been studied most, and we know a great deal about the factors that can increase your risk of contracting the disease. You'll be able to assess whether you're in a high-risk or low-risk group, and discover ways in which you can change your lifestyle and minimize your risk.

The psychological reactions to a diagnosis of cancer are complex. Breast cancer has social, emotional, and sexual consequences that will affect not only a woman's health but her relationships, her lifestyle, and her body image. A knowledgeable and well-informed woman is best placed to take an active role in her treatment, and to cultivate the mental attitude that can contribute to the defeat of the disease.

It's important for you to know that, even when a diagnosis of breast cancer is made, there are different types. Not all cancers have the same degree of invasiveness or potential for spread, so not all have a poor outlook. Try not to think of the diagnosis of breast cancer as a catastrophe. Large numbers of women live comfortably for many years after treatment. A positive state of mind is a real asset, possibly as important as some medical treatments, for we know from research done in Sweden that women who get angry at their tumors seem to live longer than women who passively accept their fate.

PIONEERS OF TREATMENT

Breast cancer is by no means a new disease; it was recorded by the ancient Egyptians and described by Hippocrates in the fifth century BC and Celsus in the first century AD. A Roman surgeon, Leonides, was known to have operated on malignant cancers of the breast at the end of the first century AD, using cautery (a hot needle) to control the bleeding and scorch any remnant of the cancer. In the same period, the Greek physician Galen set out the criteria for the surgical and medical management of breast cancer, and his guidelines were followed until the sixteenth century. We have come a long way since then. So women over the millennia have been coming to terms with breast cancer and have had to put up with much worse than we do: a letter written by the diarist Fanny Burney to her niece in the eighteenth century describes a mastectomy undertaken without any anesthetic!

THE NATURE OF BREAST CANCER

Breast cancer is a family of conditions, not a single entity. The common feature of every type, however, is that certain cells start to grow out of control. Cell growth is normally restricted to simple repair so that an organ is kept up to scratch; it is held in check by chemicals which ensure that growth is orderly and never gets out of hand. Cancer starts when the brakes on growth are taken off, or when they are no longer effective, or when cells become insensitive to them. Cell growth then becomes uncontrolled and disorderly, and the cells themselves may start to look abnormal. Because cell growth is rapid in a cancer, it absorbs a great deal of body energy. This is why cancer is often accompanied by weight loss, though this is rare in breast cancer.

TUMORS AND SPREAD

Where tissues are solid – as in the lung or the breast – fast-growing cancer cells will produce a swelling or tumor. The word *tumor* simply means a lump. Most tumors are not cancerous. They are usually benign; the growth of cells is confined to the area where the tumor starts. Tumors whose cells don't spread to other parts of the body are not fatal. In contrast, the cells that make up cancerous tumors are invasive. They spread beyond their original location – not just into adjacent tissues, but to other distant parts of the body – and as they invade tissue they destroy it.

The spread of cancer cells to the surrounding fat, downward to the muscles, or upward to the skin, is described as local spread. When cells spread further via the blood or lymphatic fluid, it is called dissemination. The original tumor is known as the primary, and tumors that arise from these cancerous cells that have spread elsewhere are called secondaries or metastases.

The rate at which cancerous cells invade or spread varies greatly; this rate determines how malignant – and therefore how dangerous – a tumor may be. To determine how aggressive cancer cells are and how far they have spread, if at all, grading and staging tests (see pp.162–66) are done. These tests also serve as a basis for deciding on treatment.

Ultrasound and blood flow velocity
Color can be added to an ultrasound image to show the rate of blood flow. The colored areas represent an increased flow rate. Although a rich blood supply to a tumor is a strong clue to malignancy, it would not on its own be a basis for a firm diagnosis.

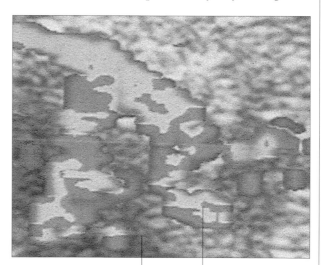

Cancer shows up as a shadowed area | Colored areas represent increased blood flow

AIDS AND BREAST CANCER

Women with AIDS do not appear to have a higher breast-cancer risk than the average woman. This interesting finding contradicts the popular belief that weakening of the immune system – whether by disease or by stressful experiences – contributes to the development of breast cancer by giving the cancerous cells more chance to take hold.

SPREAD THROUGH THE LYMPHATIC SYSTEM

Cancers of the breast often drain first into the lymph nodes in the armpits (the axillary lymph nodes), causing swelling. They may also spread to lymph nodes under the breastbone and above the collarbone. (This is why you should always include a check of your armpits and collarbone for swollen lymph nodes whenever you carry out your regular breast self-examination.) The lymphatic system (see p.40) forms a crucial part of the body's defense against infection and possibly cancer. Lymph nodes that are completely free of cancer cells are sometimes taken as a sign of a woman's high natural resistance to cancer. It may only be when this natural resistance is exhausted that the diseased cells break through into lymph nodes. If laboratory analysis discovers that the cancer has spread, this will be considered to be serious and will be reflected in the staging of the tumor, the woman's treatment, and her future outlook. The axilla will need to be treated as well as the breast (see p.180).

CANCER IN THE BLOODSTREAM

While the first sign of spread may be enlarged lymph nodes, spreading via the bloodstream is probably more important in determining the final outcome of the disease. The most recent research suggests that breast-cancer cells, or particles of them, enter the bloodstream relatively early in the course of the disease. This is why modern treatments, like chemotherapy, are aimed at eradicating cancer cells from the body *as a whole* rather than just dealing with the tumor locally. The spread of cancer through the blood probably begins with direct invasion by tumor cells of the veins that drain the breast; from there they pass into the bloodstream. These cancer "seeds" may later form secondary deposits or metastases, most commonly found in bones or the liver, lungs, or brain. It is almost always the secondary metastases that are responsible for the fatal outcome of a breast cancer.

FIBROBLASTS

Some research has centered on whether there may be some link between the character of a woman's breast tissue and her risk of developing breast cancer. Recently some researchers have suggested that it may not be the glandular elements of the breast that determine whether cells change from normal to cancerous, but cells called fibroblasts.

Fibroblasts lie among the fat and connective tissue of the breast, and produce a number of chemical messengers called growth factors. These growth factors seem to communicate with breast cancer cells, stimulating their growth and their ability to spread. Cancer cells need a rich blood supply to support their rapid growth, and fibroblasts seem to encourage the necessary formation of new blood vessels in tissues surrounding the cancer. It's probable

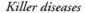

that some women's fibroblasts are more likely to support the growth of cancer cells than others, and this may help in part to explain why some breast cancers are hereditary. (For a discussion of the genetics of breast cancer, see pp.151–52).

PUTTING BREAST CANCER IN PERSPECTIVE

Breast cancer could be said to be common. In the US it affects 1 in 9 women and causes around 46,000 deaths a year; in the UK, it affects 1 in 12 women and causes around 15,000 deaths a year. This is not as frightening as it sounds; bear in mind that five times more women suffer from the disease than die from it. In a given year, of 100,000 women who live with breast cancer, 80,000 do not die. More than 70 percent of women who have operable disease will be alive and well five years after the diagnosis.

With each year you live, your chance of getting breast cancer becomes greater. Most cancers increase as people age. The likelihood of contracting the disease begins to decline only after you reach 85 or so. In evaluating the link between age and breast cancer, it is important for you to distinguish your risk as an individual woman from the risk of a whole population of women. Make sure to consider the factors other than age – for example, family history.

In statistical terms, breast cancer is the leading female cancer and accounts for almost 1 in 5 of all new cancer cases among women. In women between 35 and 55, it ranks as the commonest cause of death overall. It's only realistic, however, to put these deaths from breast cancer into perspective. For every lump in the breast that is found to be cancerous, 10 others will prove to be benign and therefore harmless. Even with cancerous lumps, 6 or 7 out of 10 will be treated without the removal of the breast, and for 3 or 4 the cause of death will be something other than cancer. If you are prepared to take the initiative so that your lump is diagnosed and treated early, you will be one of the 85 percent of women who survive for at least five years.

Although breast cancer may be the commonest cause of death in women in their 40s, in postmenopausal women – who by the year 2000 will constitute half of all women alive in the Western world – it is insignificant when compared with the number of deaths from heart disease. In this age group, the percentage of deaths due to breast cancer drops sharply, whereas the percentage of deaths due to heart disease rises quickly. Your chances of dying from a heart attack or stroke in your mid-60s are equal to those of men, whereas your chances of dying from breast cancer are probably less than half what they were when you were 50. So, although the chances of getting breast cancer increase as we age, the chances of dying from it depend on factors other than age. (Younger and older women die at about the same rates when the factors are the same.)

Killer diseases

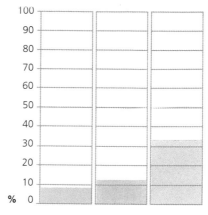

KEY

■ Breast cancer

■ Stroke

■ Cardiovascular disease

In Western women of all ages, stroke and cardiovascular disease cause many more deaths than breast cancer.

Your chances of dying from something else

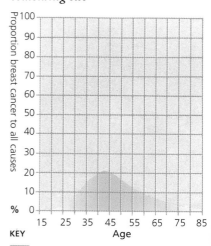

KEY

□ % deaths from other causes

■ % deaths from breast cancer

Breast cancer (represented on the graph by the green area) is the most common cause of death in women between 35 and 55. While it is more common in women over 55, it is less likely to be the cause of death in this age group.

THE GENETICS OF CANCER

A healthy cell has a well-defined shape. It is a responsible team member and only multiplies when the balance of signals is favorable. Built into cell growth, however, is the hazard of genetic mutations, or random changes. If a mutation occurs, the cell becomes damaged, and though it may look normal, it is slightly less responsive to outside signals. As genetic damage accumulates, a cell can become deaf to external messages that inhibit growth and start to show signs of malignancy. In particular, it loses its regular shape and outline and multiplies uncontrollably. Cancer probably develops because cells suffer irreversible damage to their genes. Events that cause damage to genes are called trigger factors, and those that facilitate cell growth are called promoters.

The development of a cancer cell takes time, even several lifetimes. On the other hand, it can take as little as 10 years, depending on how badly damaged the genes were when they passed from parent to child. Severely damaged genes may respond quickly to an environmental trigger, such as prolonged exposure to menstrual cycling (see p.144) in the case of breast cancer.

CANCER GENES

Normal genes that carry messages encouraging cells to multiply are called proto-oncogenes. They come in many varieties – some give cells an internal signal to multiply and others act externally by helping growth factors to stick to cells. These proto-oncogenes can be converted into cancerous forms or oncogenes. Just one change to proto-oncogenes may be enough to transform them, and some believe the damage is a result of mutations. Damage to genes that suppress tumors could also foster cancerous cell growth.

IDENTIFYING MALIGNANT CELLS

Over the past 20 years we have begun to identify many of the genes that encourage normal cells to change to cancerous ones. Every one of our cells contains 23 pairs of chromosomes, and these collectively contain all the genes that form the blueprint for human beings. When dyes are applied to them, chromosomes will take up the color in different places, showing specific regions as a series of light and dark stained bands – a kind of bar code that identifies the individual chromosome. When stained chromosomes from cancerous tumors are compared with others from normal cells, signs of genetic disarray are obvious. Some chromosomes are broken, which leads to several copies of individual chromosomes being present rather than the normal two, and whole chromosomes or segments of them may be missing altogether. Two breast cancer genes have been identified: *BRCA1* and *BRCA2* (see p.152), but there are likely to be many more.

Gene mutation
Cancer-promoting mutations in the genes of normal cells pass on the defect to future generations of cells. Later generations may acquire additional mutations until a future cell finally becomes malignant. The first woman in a family to develop breast cancer probably inherited a partially damaged gene (Stage 1 or 2). Women with a family history of breast cancer could have genes at Stage 3. Some women in breast-cancer families (see pp.151–52) carry genes that have gone all the way to Stage 4, yet, even here, cancer is not inevitable.

Normal cell

Cell no longer looks normal

1

2

Cell has become malignant

3

4

RISK AND PROTECTIVE FACTORS

Some women are more likely to get cancer of the breast than others: the risk can be connected with geographic location, particular cultures, specific personal traits, and lifestyle features. Some women inherit a susceptibility to the disease that then requires one or more environmental risk factors for breast cancer to develop. Genetic factors therefore interact with environmental factors, but unfortunately we don't know how.

We do know enough, however, to help us identify women who are at high risk. This in turn promotes early detection of breast cancer and enables some women to change their lifestyles to reduce their risk. Try to take a positive attitude and remember that some risk factors can be turned upside down to become protective factors: if having your first baby late increases the risk, you might consider having an early first child to lower your risk.

The presence of risk factors doesn't mean that a woman will inevitably develop the disease, nor does their absence guarantee that she will be free of it. In general, however, the more risk factors you have, the higher the likelihood of your developing the disease.

TYPES OF RISK

Risk is considered to be either relative or absolute. Relative risk compares a woman who has a risk factor with a woman who doesn't. This risk can vary within a single factor, however. For example, the relative risk of a woman whose mother had breast cancer is 2 – she is twice as likely to get the disease as a woman with no family history of breast cancer. But her risk increases as the age at which her mother got breast cancer decreases. So for women with a positive family history, many risk factors must be considered. (See the table of relative risks on p.150.)

Absolute risk is more precise, and denotes the number of likely cases of breast cancer in a specific number of women over a given time. The absolute risk of breast cancer is 1 woman per 1,000 per year; that is, one woman in a thousand will get breast cancer in a year.

HORMONES

A woman's hormone patterns and their fluctuations during menstruation, pregnancy, and lactation all play an important part in determining her risk of developing breast cancer. External hormones such as the contraceptive pill and hormone replacement therapy may have an effect, though this is much less. There's plenty of evidence for the effect of hormones on breast-cancer risk.

• Women with breast cancer have more female hormones than other women.

• The cells of some tumors have estrogen receptors on their surface whose presence influences the likely success of hormone treatments (see p.166).

• Breast cancer in men is rare, but in those who develop it there seems to be a link with raised estrogen levels.

• Women who for one reason or another have an artificial menopause before the age of 35 have a lower risk of breast cancer.

• Although the risk of breast cancer increases with age, the rate of this increase slows among postmenopausal women, who have lower estrogen levels than premenopausal women.

Menstruation The risk of breast cancer seems to be increased both by an early onset of menstruation (menarche) and by a late cessation of menstruation (menopause). The average Western woman's age when starting to menstruate seems to be getting earlier and the average age at menopause getting later, and this lengthening of "menstrual life" could be a contributory factor in the apparent increase in breast-cancer rates.

Researchers are coming to believe that the *total number of menstrual cycles* in a woman's lifetime determines her cancer risk. The number of menstrual cycles before the first pregnancy may be even more important, however. It is possible that the breasts are more sensitive to the action of hormones before they have fully developed – that is, before they have produced milk – and this would explain why age at first pregnancy is so important.

It is also possible that a lifetime of menstruation is an abnormal state for the human female and therefore predisposes women to develop breast cancer. In biological terms, it's only relatively recently that women stopped spending a great proportion of their reproductive life either pregnant or breastfeeding. In addition, it's only this century that women in any numbers have lived long enough to reach menopause at all. The average Western girl now starts to menstruate before the age of 12, but will then wait until she is 25 or 26 years old to have her first baby, exposing her to almost 14 years of continuous menstrual cycling before her first pregnancy. This does not happen in many other cultures. A teenage African girl may not start menstruating until she's 17 or 18 because she's undernourished, and may then become pregnant almost at once, saving her from many years of exposure to cyclical estrogens.

Pregnancy Having babies undoubtedly protects women against breast cancer; this may be because it saves a woman from being exposed to cyclical estrogens for nine months. The major protection seems to be conferred by the first pregnancy, which must be carried to term to be protective; a first pregnancy that ends in abortion or miscarriage does not have any protective effect.

MENSTRUAL LIFE AND CANCER RISK

Your "menstrual life" links three important breast-cancer risk factors: age at first period, age at menopause, and number of pregnancies. Even small differences between women can add up to significant differences in overall risk.

Joan		Liz	
Age at menopause	52	*Age at menopause*	48
Less age at first period	-12	*Less age at first period*	-14
Less time spent pregnant (years)	-1½	*Less time spent pregnant (years)*	-3
Total years' exposure to estrogen	38½	*Total years' exposure to estrogen*	31

Not having children and having a first baby late in life both seem to increase the chances of developing breast cancer. For women who have their first child after the age of 30 the risk of breast cancer is about twice that of women who have their first child before the age of 20. Women who remain childless are at increased risk, and this may partly explain why infertility in older women is linked to breast cancer. Surprisingly, women who have their first child after 35 appear to be at an even higher risk than women who have no children.

The contraceptive pill The oral contraceptive pill was introduced 30 years ago and has been used by about 150 million women. Huge long-term research studies have not uncovered any substantial increased risk of breast cancer in women who take the pill. Breast cancer is fairly common, as is the practice of taking the pill, so if breast cancer develops in a woman who is on the pill we can't assume the two are related – it might have happened anyway. The pill has probably been more closely studied than any other medication in the twentieth century, and most doctors believe that, for a woman who is sexually active and for whom effective and convenient contraception is important, the benefits almost certainly outweigh any risks. Only those pills that contain estrogen remain at all controversial. The progesterone-only pill, or "mini-pill," carries no risk at all of breast cancer.

If the pill is linked to breast cancer at all, it is more likely that it acts as a promoter than as a trigger; that is, it provides the conditions that allow cells to multiply rather than actually causing the genetic mutations that make them do so. (While it's very unlikely that the use of the pill could alter the growth rate or the behavior of a tumor, most doctors would nevertheless advise using the progesterone-only pill or some other method of contraception after treatment of breast cancer.)

Among women who have a family history of breast cancer, the pill may cause a slight increase in risk, and women who start to take the pill when they are very young and continue to take it for longer than eight years before they first become pregnant also have a small increased risk. But this risk has to be kept in perspective. It is something like a 3 in 1,000 chance of developing breast cancer under the age of 35, compared with 2 in 1,000 for women who have never used the pill – considerably less than the risk of being run over by a car while crossing the road!

Against these very small increases in risk we have to weigh the fact that the pill has a protective effect against ovarian cancer. For a woman at risk for ovarian cancer, this protective effect would outweigh the breast cancer risk. Some studies have also shown a reduction in benign breast disease among pill users – but there is little data available to support this.

Hormone replacement therapy Menopausal symptoms have been successfully treated with hormone replacement therapy (HRT) for more than 50 years. There has been no dramatic increase in breast cancer, however, since the use of HRT became fairly widespread some two decades ago, suggesting that any

Family history and risk

25 times normal risk

Mother with bilateral breast cancer under 35

Mother and sister with breast cancer

Sister with bilateral breast cancer under 40

Sister with bilateral breast cancer under 50

First-degree relative (mother or sister) with breast cancer

Second-degree relative (aunt or grandmother) with breast cancer

Normal risk

The more relatives a woman has with breast cancer, and the younger they are when they get the disease, the higher her own risk becomes.

risk is very small. Most researchers in this field agree that in the first 10 years of use there is no increased risk associated with HRT. After that time there may be a very small increased risk, though this is largely confined to certain groups of women who already have risk factors, such as those with a positive family history or atypical hyperplasia (see p.155). For the average healthy woman, it would appear that the use of HRT does not increase breast-cancer risk any more than having a first baby after the age of 30 does.

As with the contraceptive pill, there are also benefits to be weighed against any possible risk. HRT has a protective effect against cancers of the lung, colon, ovary, and cervix. It also protects against heart disease, the major killer of women, and osteoporosis. Women on HRT who develop breast cancer usually have a less invasive form of cancer. They tend to be estrogen- and progesterone-receptor-positive (see p.166) when the cancer is diagnosed, making the response to hormone treatment more likely. Women who develop breast cancer after having taken HRT for eight years have an improved survival rate. Finally, women who have used HRT seem to have a lower mortality rate at any age from any cause than those who have not.

HRT may be offered to women at high risk of developing breast cancer but must be carefully monitored. Even for women who have had breast cancer, HRT needn't be ruled out as long as there is careful follow-up from a doctor who is expert in this field. If you fall into this category, you should talk it over with a gynecologist as well as a cancer specialist.

FAMILY HISTORY

A family history of breast cancer is a strong risk factor in itself; it also makes all other risk factors potentially more dangerous. The increase in risk depends on how close the relative is and on how many relatives have had breast cancer. The affected relative can come from either the maternal or paternal side of the family, or she may have developed breast cancer under the age of 50; risk increases still further if *two* female relatives are affected.

A woman whose mother developed cancer in both breasts before the age of 35, for instance, has a 50 percent chance of developing breast cancer herself. This familial susceptibility to breast cancer is now known to be related to two genes, labeled *BRCA1* and *BRCA2* (see p.152). Being born into a "breast-cancer family" (see pp.151–52) carries the greatest risk, and it's important to identify these high-risk women.

AGE

Given that environmental factors can react with a genetic predisposition to trigger the growth of breast cancer, it stands to reason that the longer a woman lives the more likely she is to be exposed to these environmental triggers, and the higher her risk of developing breast cancer. This supposition is borne out by the statistics: about half of all breast cancers occur in women aged 50–64, with a further 30 percent in women over 70. This means that 80 percent of breast cancers occur over the age of 50.

GEOGRAPHY

The frequency of breast cancer varies widely throughout the world. In the Western world, for example, it's one of the most common cancers, but it's much less common in Asia, Eastern Europe, and among black women in Africa. Determining why this is so is not a simple matter, however. Environment, race, diet, climate, patterns of infection, cultural influences, birth control methods, age of first pregnancy, and the popularity of breast-feeding are all possible contributors to the geographic pattern. Women of higher socioeconomic status are more prone to breast cancer, and this may imply that there are dietary and social factors at work.

Breast cancer seems to single out white women living in colder climates in highly industrialized societies, and it's the Western lifestyle that is largely to blame. Women from low-risk areas such as Japan (which has one of the lowest rates of breast cancer in the world) who move to higher-risk countries such as the US climb into a higher risk group for breast cancer. Environmental factors therefore seem to be stronger than racial or inherited factors. There is even evidence that shows rates of breast cancer increasing as countries become more industrialized.

The picture is further complicated by the fact that breast cancer behaves differently in different places. Not only do Japanese women who live in Japan have a low incidence of breast cancer; when they get it, it seems to occur in younger women than in the West, which suggests that there may be some genetic factors that are independent of environmental risks.

RADIATION

We have known for some time that high doses of radiation can promote the development of breast cancer. In the past, women who received high-dose chest X-rays to check on treatment for tuberculosis ran an increased risk of developing cancer. Japanese women who were exposed to enormously high doses of radiation from the atomic bombs at Hiroshima and Nagasaki are still developing breast cancer at higher rates than other Japanese women of the same age living elsewhere.

The higher the dose of X-rays and the larger the number of exposures, the greater the risk. Furthermore, there seems to be no lower limit at which we can say that the risk disappears. This is why radiation is always handled with great care by doctors and nurses.

BREASTFEEDING

Breastfeeding does seem to protect against breast cancer, though pregnancy is more important; early pregnancy (see above) is protective whether a woman breastfeeds or bottlefeeds. Evidence from the animal kingdom shows that lactation is protective: dairy cows, who lactate constantly, are never found to develop cancer of the udders. An interesting phenomenon, though probably apocryphal, can be observed among Hong Kong boat women. They suckle their babies almost entirely from the left breast so that they can keep their

Incidence of breast cancer
The list below shows the relative positions of 24 countries in a "league table" of breast cancer rates, with Western Europe at the top of the league with the highest rates.

1 England and Wales
2 Denmark
3 Scotland
4 N. Ireland
5 Netherlands
6 Belgium
7 Switzerland
8 New Zealand
9 Canada
10 Germany
11 US
12 Hungary
13 Czechoslovakia
14 Australia
15 Argentina
16 France
17 Norway
18 Sweden
19 Portugal
20 Poland
21 Bulgaria
22 Greece
23 Hong Kong
24 Japan

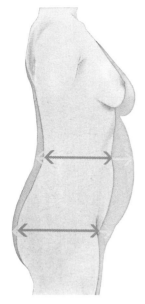

Premenopausal figure: waist smaller than hips, healthy pattern

Postmenopausal figure: waist larger than hips, high-risk pattern

Obesity and risk
The pattern of obesity is important in determining risk, since deposits of fat on the waist and stomach confer a higher risk. This unhealthy fat pattern is characteristic of postmenopausal women and is related to increased risk of heart disease.

right hand free for rowing their boats. When they do develop breast cancer, which is rare, it's more often in the right breast – the breast that has not been used in breastfeeding. Some evidence from US studies suggests that breastfeeding even for a very short time is protective. As breastfeeding confers such a substantial protective effect, and as it is available to all women who give birth, it's astonishing that more women don't do it. I would urge all women to consider breastfeeding, even for as short a time as a couple of weeks.

DIET

The Western diet is constantly cited as a risk factor for breast cancer, but the evidence is pretty thin. The original connection came from an observation that dietary fat can cause breast tumors in rats. Such evidence can't be directly applied to human beings, but it was an interesting lead. Studies of total fat intake, however, have not found that women with breast cancer consume a significantly higher amount than women without; the relationship may reflect total caloric intake rather than fat intake alone. The breast cancer risk seems more influenced by obesity than by fat consumption.

An extensive experiment is under way in the US. Women who have reduced their animal fat consumption to no more than 20 percent of total calories will be compared with an age-matched group of women on a Westernized diet, which typically takes about 40 percent of its calories from animal fat. Any differences in breast cancer rates between the two groups will support the theory that animal fats constitute a risk factor.

Fat consumption may not be a straightforward link. Those who eat a diet high in fat tend to eat less fruit and vegetables, and it could be that the risk is due to a deficiency of fiber in the diet rather than an excess of fat. Very recent evidence suggests that a diet rich in cereals and vegetables may protect against breast cancer. Fiber is thought to influence estrogen metabolism, and some vitamin derivatives may have a protective effect, particularly vitamin E and beta-carotene, a form of vitamin A.

One recent European study has shown that a soy-rich diet will lengthen the menstrual cycle by two or three days. Over a lifetime this would mean significantly fewer cycles, having a beneficial effect with regard to breast cancer (see p.144). The active components of soy are isoflavones, which have a strong estrogenic effect.

OBESITY

Overweight women have a higher risk of dying from breast cancer than do their thinner sisters. It used to be thought this was because cancers were difficult to discover in larger breasts and so were found at a more advanced stage; this is not so. In fact, fat cells manufacture additional estrogen, leading to excessive exposure, particularly in postmenopausal women.

The pattern of obesity seems to be important in defining cancer risk. When fat is concentrated around the trunk, giving a ratio between waist and hip measurements of greater than 1 (an "apple shape"), cancer risk is higher than in women who retain a well-defined waist with bigger hips ("pear shapes"). This pattern of obesity is linked with a number of diseases, such as heart disease in men. It's a common fat distribution among postmenopausal and infertile women, in whom breast cancer rates are higher than average.

ALCOHOL

Excessive alcohol intake increases a woman's risk of developing breast cancer in the long term, because alcohol can interfere with estrogen metabolism in the liver. Both alcohol and estrogen are broken down in the liver and, after many years of exposure to alcohol, the liver loses its ability to metabolize estrogen. This results in increased levels of estrogen in the blood, a factor we know to increase the risk of breast cancer.

This link with alcohol is not a great risk and must be kept in perspective: if a thousand women over the age of 30 drank moderately for two years, there would be one extra case of breast cancer among them. On the other hand, moderate alcohol intake reduces the number of cases of heart disease and can improve the quality of life. Research does not suggest that the majority of women need to alter their drinking habits, so it's up to the individual woman. If, however, you already fall into a high-risk group for some other reason, you should consider keeping your alcohol consumption low.

VIRUSES

There are many instances among animals, particularly in cats and mice, of a connection between viruses and the development of cancer. In a certain strain of mice, breast cancer is so common that it can be transmitted from mothers to daughters. Breast milk from these mice has been found to contain particles of a virus that can create cancerous changes in normal body cells. This is not true of human breast milk. There is, however, an isolated community of Iranian women who have a much higher chance than normal of developing breast cancer in their lifetime – as high as 1 in 5. Their breast milk contains particles similar to the breast-cancer virus found in mice. No other similar group of women has so far been located anywhere in the world, and as yet no study has been done to compare breast cancer rates in women who were breastfed and women who were bottlefed as babies.

SMOKING

Rates of breast cancer are lower in smokers than in nonsmokers, though this can never be advocated as a reason for smoking – the risk of dying from a smoking-related disease far outweighs that of dying from breast cancer.

It is thought that smoking exerts an anti-estrogenic effect, accelerating the onset of menopause; smokers typically reach menopause three to four years earlier than nonsmokers. Smokers tend to be thinner than nonsmokers; we know that estrogens are manufactured in the fatty tissues and that obesity is a risk factor for breast cancer. Smokers also have fewer incidences of benign breast disease than nonsmokers, and this could partly explain the reduced risk.

The protective effect of smoking is greater among postmenopausal than premenopausal women, and seems to operate only as long as you continue smoking. As soon as you stop, the protection is lost.

As yet we don't fully understand why smoking has this anti-estrogenic effect. It could be due to suppression of estrogen production, inhibition of estrogen activity, or promotion of estrogen breakdown. One study has found that women who smoke have higher levels of male sex hormones, such as testosterone, which has anti-estrogenic properties.

WHAT YOU CAN DO

Factors like your family history or age at menopause are beyond your control, but there are some aspects of your lifestyle that you can change to make a difference to your risk of breast cancer.

• Restrict the fat intake in your diet and increase your fiber intake by eating plenty of whole-grain cereals, fruit, and vegetables.

• Enjoy alcohol only in moderation.

• Keep your body fat down with a balanced diet and regular exercise.

• If you have children, breastfeed – the longer the better.

Comparison of risk
Some factors, such as age at first menstrual period, increase risk only a little; others, such as family history, increase it far more. When referring to this chart, remember that the lowest possible risk has a score of 1.0.

RISK FACTOR	LOWEST RISK		SLIGHT INCREASE		MODERATE INCREASE	
Age at first menstrual period	*16 years (late)*	*1.0*	*15 years (late)*	*1.1*		
			11–14 years (normal)	*1.3*		
Age at menopause	*Before 45*	*1.0*	*45–54*	*1.4*	*Over 55*	*2.1*
Age at birth of first child	*Before 20*	*1.0*	*20–29*	*1.45*	*Over 30 years or no children*	*1.9*
Family history	*None*	*1.0*	*Mother affected before age 60*	*2.0*	*Two first-degree relatives affected (i.e., mother and sister)*	*4.0–6.0*
			Mother affected after age 60	*1.4*		
Benign breast disease	*None*	*1.0*	*Increase in number of cells*	*2.0*	*Atypical hyperplasia (see p.155)*	*4.5*
Alcohol intake	*None*	*1.0*	*1 drink a day*	*1.4*	*3 drinks a day*	*2.0*
			2 drinks a day	*1.7*		
Radiation exposure	*No special exposure*	*1.0*	*Repeated X-rays*	*1.5–2.0*	*Atomic bomb*	*3.0*
Oral contraceptives	*Never used or no longer used*	*1.0*	*Currently used*	*1.5*	*Prolonged use before pregnancy*	*2.0*
HRT	*Never used or no longer used*	*1.0*	*Currently used all ages*	*1.4*	*Used longer than 10 years or currently used over 60*	*2.1*

BREAST-CANCER FAMILIES

A single first-degree relative (that is, mother or sister) with breast cancer doubles anyone's risk of cancer, but in breast-cancer families the risks are even greater. A breast-cancer family is one in which the risk of developing breast cancer is determined almost totally by family history, and appears to be independent of other risk factors, except atypical hyperplasia (see p.155).

Breast cancer families, though quite rare, have been studied for more than two millennia and were first reported in Roman medical literature of 100 AD. In the 1860s, an American doctor, Paul Broca, described many instances of breast cancer in combination with bowel cancer in several generations of his wife's family. He was describing what we now call hereditary breast cancer (HBC). The word hereditary means that the cancer runs through a family, affecting successive generations of women. The pattern of inheritance nearly always suggests that the hereditary factor is extremely strong. The factor responsible has been narrowed down to one or two genes (see p.152), and because it's so strong we call it a dominant gene. Although hereditary breast cancer puts women at very high risk, it accounts for only a small proportion of all cases of breast cancer – between 5 and 10 percent.

KEY

◯ Male

◉ Female

⊗ Deceased

◉ Breast cancer

A RIGOROUS APPROACH

There are several important features of HBC that profoundly affect treatment. The first is the early age of onset. Breast cancer is more common in older women as a rule, with an average age of 62 years among women affected, but in breast-cancer families the average age is 44. Second, there is often more than one tumor in the breast. Finally, the cancer may affect both breasts.

A family history of breast cancer
When one sister contracted breast cancer (a great-aunt and an aunt having died of cancer), her three younger sisters sought expert advice. One of the sisters, diagnosed early with breast cancer, was successfully treated. Both other sisters were found to be clear.

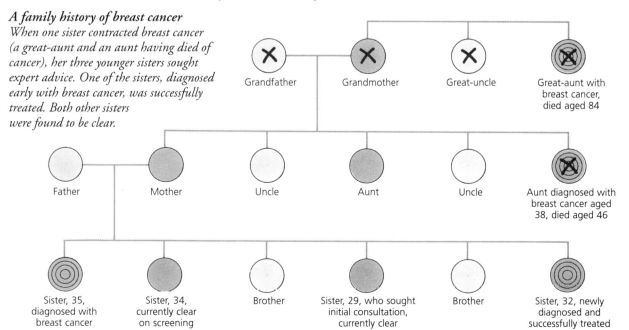

Grandfather — Grandmother — Great-uncle — Great-aunt with breast cancer, died aged 84

Father — Mother — Uncle — Aunt — Uncle — Aunt diagnosed with breast cancer aged 38, died aged 46

Sister, 35, diagnosed with breast cancer — Sister, 34, currently clear on screening — Brother — Sister, 29, who sought initial consultation, currently clear — Brother — Sister, 32, newly diagnosed and successfully treated

These three characteristics have an enormous bearing on how doctors view familial breast cancer. Women who belong to these families must be identified and forewarned that they are in danger of developing breast cancer early and in both breasts. Any woman who is aware of her risk should seek advice from a breast center while still in her teens or early 20s. Because of the aggressive nature of this cancer, doctors are more likely to be open to the idea of prophylactic mastectomy (see p.153) with reconstruction (see p.189), if you really want to go that far, though medically it's hard to justify when inheritance of the gene can not, as yet, be proved

The shadow cast by the hereditary pattern of HBC falls on all aspects of managing it. Monitoring the health of the breasts must be rigorous and scrupulous, with regular checkups, mammograms, ultrasonic scans where appropriate, and biopsies of any suspicious changes.

IDENTIFYING WOMEN AT RISK

At present the most important tool for both doctor and patient is a thorough family history. Unfortunately we have no way of testing for the precise genes and chromosomes associated with HBC and identifying vulnerable women before the cancer appears, though there is hope that such tests will become possible in the next few years. Until then, a careful family pedigree and close surveillance, with frequent physical examinations and mammograms, are our best weapons. There has been much controversy surrounding the time for starting mammographic screening. The problem with mammograms in younger women is that the breasts are more dense (see p.48) and cancers are difficult to pick up. Several studies have shown, though, that early detection is possible, and it's certainly worthwhile in breast-cancer families.

Careful surveillance of cancer families is essential. This is best done by gathering the female members of the family together to explain how cancers can run through generations in a family, offering counseling, and subjecting each woman to vigorous screening and testing to detect any cancers early.

BREAST CANCER GENES

A gene responsible for inherited breast cancer (*BRCA1*) was identified in 1994 by Dr. Mark Skolnick in Salt Lake City, Utah. Research on a second gene (*BRCA2*) is under way, and more are likely to be found. *BRCA1* and *BRCA2* are probably responsible for more than half the cases of inherited breast cancer. A woman with either gene has about an 80 percent lifetime risk of contracting breast cancer, falling to 70 percent after the age of 50. The genes can be passed on by either parent; there is a fifty–fifty chance that children will inherit them.

At the moment no gene test is commercially available – there are many possible gene mutations, presenting complex problems for testing – but it is likely that within the next five years, women from breast-cancer families could be offered a test. Women found to carry the genes would then have the options of increased monitoring to detect cancer early, including annual mammography from age 35, tamoxifen therapy, or preventive surgery.

PREVENTIVE MEASURES

An overview of breast-cancer risk factors (see pp.143–50) shows that there are some factors we can control to reduce our risk – notably diet, alcohol intake, an early first child, and, for women who have children, breastfeeding. For women at very high risk, however, some kind of prevention in the form of hormone treatment or surgery may be advisable.

TAMOXIFEN

A complex drug with estrogenic and anti-estrogenic properties, tamoxifen was first used in the treatment of breast cancer and is now being studied as a way of preventing it among high-risk women, particularly those with a strong family history where breast cancer may appear at an early age (see pp.151–52). Tamoxifen is used to treat women who already have breast cancer; not only does it reduce the risk of recurrence and improve mortality rates, but in the long term it also reduces by half the risk of getting cancer in the other breast, a cause of great concern for women with a family history.

Just as fibroblast growth factors (see p.140) promote breast cancer, other growth factors suppress it. The production of suppressor growth factors is stimulated by tamoxifen – one reason it might help prevent breast cancer.

Because of its anti-estrogenic action, tamoxifen has side effects when taken for long periods, causing menopausal symptoms and an early onset of menopause or possibly a slightly increased risk of uterine cancer. It is also not recommended after thrombosis. You may find these risks worth tolerating, however, because tamoxifen has life-saving properties other than reducing the risk of breast cancer. It seems to protect against heart attacks – in a recent study in Scotland it led to a significant reduction in deaths from heart disease – and to prevent the onset of osteoporosis.

PROPHYLACTIC MASTECTOMY

If you are at high risk of developing breast cancer, you may have seen your mother or sister die from the disease and may seek mastectomy as a way of preventing it in yourself. Prophylactic (preventive) mastectomy is a surgical operation that aims to reduce the risk of breast cancer by removing as much of the breast tissue as possible. Reconstruction may be carried out at the same time or later to rebuild the breast. In such a case a subcutaneous mastectomy – an operation where the breast tissue is removed from beneath the skin and an implant inserted, leaving the nipple and areola intact – is not an option. The operation *must* be a total mastectomy – anything else is not justifiable. If your doctor suggests a subcutaneous mastectomy, question its reliability and usefulness and get a second opinion.

This is a controversial operation. Many doctors are loath to remove healthy breast tissue when cancer may never develop. Also crucial is whether the operation is effective enough in preventing breast cancer when powerful non-surgical treatments could accomplish the same goal. When contemplating prophylactic mastectomy, you must remember that there is no guarantee that cancer will be prevented. For these reasons, you will be considered eligible to have both breasts removed only if you fulfill the following strict criteria:

• an unarguable family history and an estimated 50 percent chance of getting breast cancer.

• your clear understanding that if you run a 50 percent chance of carrying the high-risk gene you also have a 50 percent chance of not carrying the gene and thus being at normal risk for breast cancer.

• the presence of additional factors that would raise the risk above 50 percent, such as two sisters being affected or atypical hyperplasia (see p.155).

Breasts that are difficult to examine clinically and radiographically, plus severe cancer phobia, would also be taken into consideration. You should decide to have a prophylactic mastectomy only after careful discussion of your precise risk, details of the operation, and the likely results with a specialist breast surgeon and the other members of the breast management team. Even better would be counseling by two doctors who can evaluate your risk factors and their implications. Finally, you should also consult close family and friends. Most women, when advised that they have a chance of not carrying the high-risk gene, opt for intensive follow-up rather than surgery.

The majority of women at high risk are monitored most effectively by breast self-examination and regular physical examinations and mammograms. In addition, the use of fine-needle aspiration (see p.127) is decreasing the need for open biopsy if a breast lump should ever occur, and biopsy is available for any suspicious breast areas that may arise.

MAKING THE DECISION

Pros
• Although there is no definite evidence to prove that prophylactic mastectomy reduces a woman's chance of getting cancer, it probably does, as long as the operation is a total mastectomy.
• The operation certainly reduces painful symptoms and tender lumpiness in the breast as part of the menstrual cycle, though mastalgia alone would never be a reason for mastectomy.
• For women who cannot live normal lives for fear of breast cancer, it can provide a new lease of life.
• Modern surgical procedures mean that the breasts can be reconstructed.
• Careful follow-up increases the probability of finding your cancer at a very early stage.

Cons
• There are the risks of general anesthesia and complications including bleeding, infection, skin loss, contracture (see p.114), and damage to the implant. Also, the nipple is removed.
• Complications can occur if an abdominal flap is used for reconstruction (see p.179).
• The reconstructed breast is rarely as attractive as the original breast, and there may be permanent scars and loss of sensation.
• More than one operation may be needed to achieve the best results or manage complications.
• There's no guarantee that cancer will be prevented: not all breast tissue is removed, and any that is left behind is a potential site for breast cancer.

NONINVASIVE CANCER

The glands and ducts that make up the breast lobules are in a state of growth, development, and shrinkage during a woman's fertile life (see pp.116–17). Overgrowth of cells, or hyperplasia, may occur in any part of the lobes or ducts. The word *hyperplasia* without qualification describes a benign condition, although it carries a small increase in cancer risk. In some hyperplasias, however, the cells become somewhat unusual or atypical. This is referred to as atypical hyperplasia, and has a moderate chance of turning into a localized cancer. (A woman with a family history of breast cancer who gets atypical hyperplasia moves into a very high risk group indeed.)

At the far end of the atypical hyperplasia spectrum comes actual cancer, but at first at least, it is the noninvasive cancer "in situ." This term is used for patterns of cell growth that are confined to the duct or lobule where they originated but that carry a high risk of becoming invasive.

UNDERSTANDING HYPERPLASIA

In assessing hyperplasia, there are several features that doctors look at to decide whether the condition is benign or whether there is a risk of cancer, including the rate at which the cells are dividing, the way they are organized, and the features of the cells themselves, such as their shape or the size of the nuclei. The condition that most concerns doctors is atypical hyperplasia, which exhibits some but not all the features of cancer in terms of both the appearance of the cells and their patterns of growth.

PRE-INVASIVE DISEASE

As cell growth proceeds from hyperplasia, which is benign, toward malignancy, it reaches an in-between stage – cancer "in situ." The words *in situ* are Latin and mean that the cancer is confined to its place of origin. This is a crucial distinction to make, because these cancers by definition are not invasive, and they are seldom fatal. There are two kinds: ductal carcinoma in situ (DCIS) and lobular carcinoma in situ (LCIS).

In situ carcinomas are confined to the duct or lobule in which they start growing, and rarely invade the surrounding breast. A true lump is often difficult to detect, and unless there is some other symptom such as nipple discharge, the majority of these lumps are only picked up through screening mammograms, when the characteristic tiny Y-shaped calcifications of DCIS are seen.

PROGRESS OF HYPERPLASIA

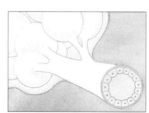

Normal duct
The cells lining the ducts and lobes multiply only under strictly regulated conditions and in response to specific signals.

Stage 1   Stage 2

Stage 3   Stage 4

1 *Hyperplasia*
The cells multiply more than necessary, creating a harmless excess that builds up inside the duct.

2 *Atypical hyperplasia*
The cells lose their normal appearance and are called "atypical." This is still a benign condition.

3 *Carcinoma in situ*
The atypical cells fill up the duct, forming a carcinoma. They are not invasive, however.

4 *Invasive carcinoma*
The cells break out of the duct and spread to the surrounding tissues. This is a true invasive cancer.

In situ cancers sometimes pose a problem for treatment because it is not known how many may progress to invasive cancer, nor how long they take to do so. Nor has one approach to the treatment of DCIS and LCIS been proved to be substantially better than any other.

Because of the risk that an in situ DCIS cancer may turn invasive, preventive mastectomy may be an option. Most doctors, however, would probably adopt the compromise of a wide excision to remove the cancerous tissue and a watch policy, with mastectomy later if necessary. Ultimately the choice of treatment depends on a woman's individual risk, whether she has a family history of breast cancer, whether there is calcification in her breast lesion (see p.158), and her age when it is discovered.

LOBULAR CARCINOMA IN SITU (LCIS)

LCIS in itself does not develop into cancer, but it is useful as a marker, showing that a woman is at risk of developing DCIS. This explains why breast cancer in women who have been diagnosed with LCIS doesn't always develop in the same spot as the LCIS, or even in the same breast. Because of this, removing the affected lobe will not reduce the risk, so the woman with LCIS is in the same position as other women at high risk – that is, she has the options of either having both breasts removed or having close follow-up, with regular breast self-examination, medical checks, and mammograms. Most women opt for the latter.

DUCTAL CARCINOMA IN SITU (DCIS)

DCIS represents the extreme end of the spectrum of hyperplasia (see p.155); a woman with DCIS has 11 times the normal risk of developing invasive cancer. It is most common in breast ducts adjacent to an established cancer – often being found when a cancerous lump is removed – and is therefore nearly always treated by some form of breast surgery. DCIS tends to fall into two distinct types: focal (occurring in only one spot in the breast) and multicentric (in several parts of the breast), with little tendency for the first to proceed to the second.

In situ cancers
The cells in the slide of LCIS (right) are uniform, being small and round. The alveoli or glands can be seen but are abnormal because they're not hollow. In the slide of DCIS (far right), a single alveolus or gland is visible. The cells are not uniform in shape, have no recognizable structure, and appear to be growing to fill the space inside the gland. Some of the nuclei inside the cells are dark and sinister in appearance.

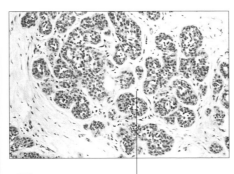

LCIS

Abnormally dark nucleus

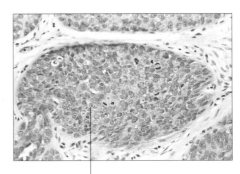

DCIS

Alveolus or gland

For multicentric DCIS, total mastectomy will be recommended. If mammograms do not show clearly which type is present, however, a wide excision of the lump plus a margin of normal tissue will be performed, or the whole quadrant of the affected breast will be removed. The tissue that has been removed is then examined under a microscope, and, if the DCIS is found to have more than one focus, total mastectomy will be performed after discussion with the patient.

If the original area of DCIS is the only focus in all the material removed, a further surgical procedure may not be recommended. Follow-up is crucial, however, because of the increased risk of invasive cancer, and should take the form of monthly self-examination (see p.60), yearly clinical examination by a doctor, and two-yearly mammography. Radiotherapy has also proven to be effective in decreasing local recurrence of DCIS, and is therefore recommended.

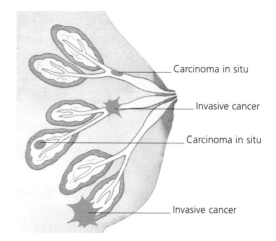

Carcinoma in situ

Invasive cancer

Carcinoma in situ

Invasive cancer

Sites of cancer
Breast cancer can arise in either the lobes or, more rarely, the milk ducts. If it is noninvasive and remains confined to the lobe or duct, it is termed "carcinoma in situ." Once it spreads to the surrounding tissue, it is a true invasive cancer.

TRUE CANCER

As a rule, breast cancers arise from the cells that line the ducts or lobules. The most frequent form is known as ductal carcinoma, because it was originally thought to arise from the milk ducts. It is now recognized, however, that both this type and the less common lobular carcinoma usually arise in the breast lobule. All other forms of breast cancer are rare. Both ductal and lobular carcinomas can be pre-invasive (in situ, see above) or invasive.

Invasive ductal carcinoma Ductal carcinomas comprise over 80 percent of all detected breast cancers. The first symptom is generally a new, hard, ill-defined lump within the breast. As the tumor spreads along the ligaments of Cooper (see p.38) between the breast lobes, it pulls on the overlying skin, creating a characteristic dimpling effect. Extreme skin pitting, known as *peau d'orange* because the skin resembles orange peel, is a serious sign. If the tumor spreads along the ducts it will pull on and eventually invert the nipple; this is why a new inversion of the nipple should always prompt you to visit your doctor, though it can also be caused by duct ectasia (see p.132), which is a benign condition. The lymph nodes under the armpits may be involved, and as the tumor spreads it may involve the underlying muscles. The smaller and less advanced the cancer is at the time of diagnosis, the better the outlook for the patient (see pp.162–65).

Invasive lobular carcinoma Lobular carcinomas account for about 10 percent of all breast cancers and behave in a very similar way to ductal cancers. The main difference, however, is that lobular carcinomas may spread diffusely rather than forming a discrete tumor.

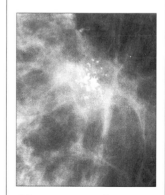

Mammogram of DCIS
An in situ cancer will not be felt as a lump, but may be detected by mammography. On this mammogram, the cluster of white dots in the middle are calcifications that signify a ductal carcinoma in situ.

DETECTION AND DIAGNOSIS

Mammography is your lifeline. Routine mammographic screening can cut the death rate from breast cancer by 20–30 percent. For instance, DCIS becomes invasive in 50–75 percent of cases within five years, so early detection is vital. Mammography can detect cancers less than $^1/_4$ inch (0.5 centimeters) across, whereas a lump cannot be felt by you or your doctor until it has grown to about $^1/_2$ inch (1 centimeter). Since the early 1980s, screening has resulted in a decrease in the average size of breast tumors diagnosed in American women. In the UK, 30 to 50 percent of detected tumors now measure less than $^3/_4$ inch (2 centimeters) when they are first diagnosed; 20 years ago the proportion was only 5–10 percent.

There are drawbacks, however. Some doctors are concerned about the number of marginal abnormalities detected by mammography, which may then be treated when they should probably be left alone. If doctors operate on women as if they had invasive breast cancer – perhaps even performing mastectomy – there is the possibility that women will undergo unnecessary surgery. Despite these questions it must be remembered that mammography is the best screening tool we have for the detection of breast cancer, and the only screening method for malignancy, the value of which has been proved by rigorous clinical trials.

SPECIAL CASES FOR SCREENING

The American Cancer Society recommends annual mammograms in all women after the age of 40; the incidence of breast cancer is lower in younger women and mammography is less efficient when breast tissue is more dense. Women between the ages of 18 and 40 should also examine their breasts monthly, and have them examined once a year by a physician. In special cases, however, screening should be carried out at an earlier age.

US guidelines for a woman with a first-degree relative who develops pre-menopausal breast cancer are that she be screened every two years, starting when she is ten years younger than the age at which her relative developed breast cancer. Women diagnosed with atypical hyperplasia (see p.155) are also advised to have a mammogram every year.

IDENTIFYING CANCER

Mammography does not only reveal cancer. Benign lumps, which have rounded smooth edges and a halo of healthy fat around them, can also be seen. Cancerous lumps, on the other hand, are more dense at the center than at the edges, which are often irregular. Mammography may also be able to show other changes such as skin thickening, or tethering and distortion of breast tissue around a lump. A deposit of calcium particles (calcification) may show up as white dots. In a benign lump, the calcification appears as relatively large blobs, but with cancer it has a characteristic fine speckled appearance which to an experienced radiologist is virtually diagnostic of malignancy.

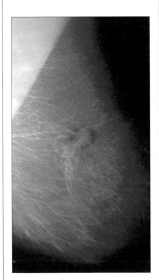

Cancerous tumor
The area colored red in the center of this mammogram is a cancer. The uneven "starburst" outline is typical of an invasive tumor.

DIAGNOSIS

Doctors use many investigative techniques and skills in order to come to as specific a diagnosis as possible when a woman finds a lump in her breast. The initial sequence of tests varies, depending on whether the lump has been found by the woman herself or detected on a mammogram, in which case it may be too small to feel. In all cases, however, a sample of cells or tissue will have to be examined under a microscope to determine whether the lump is malignant; if it is, further tests will be carried out to assess the precise origin of the tumor, its grade, and its stage (see pp.162–64).

CLINICAL DIAGNOSIS

The doctor will first look at your breasts while you sit with your hands by your side and then with your arms raised above your head, so that he or she can observe any asymmetry between the breasts, nipple retraction, difference in level between the nipples, or skin dimpling. If you've been doing regular breast self-examination, you'll be able to confirm which of these features are new and which you have observed in the past. You'll then be asked to lie back while the doctor examines your breasts carefully, feeling each quadrant of both breasts with the flat of the hand. The aim is to decide whether there is an obvious, discrete lump or if the breasts are just generally lumpy. The doctor will then check the underarm region on both sides for any lumps caused by swollen lymph nodes, and the area above the collarbone (also to check for swollen lymph nodes), the abdomen, and the chest.

If your symptoms are lumpiness of the breasts or pain or both, but no obvious new discrete lump is found on examination, further management will depend on your age. If you are under the age of 40, cancer is unlikely, and you may be asked to return in six weeks. If you still have pain from a lumpy breast, then treatment may be advised (see p.124). If you are over 40, a mammogram may be advised to ensure that no hidden cancer is present. If this shows no evidence of malignancy, you can be reassured and offered treatment for your symptoms if necessary. If there is any suspicion of cancerous pattern on the mammogram, FNAC will be advised (see p.127), and perhaps further tests, depending on the result of the FNAC.

Discharge from the nipple will be tested to see if it contains blood, as this is not always obvious to the naked eye, and the doctor will note whether the discharge comes from a single duct or many. Nipple discharge is usually associated with benign conditions (see pp.133–34), but in rare cases a bloodless discharge from either single or multiple ducts may require further investigation to rule out cancer. Your doctor will need to perform a biopsy, since laboratory tests of the discharge are too inaccurate to rely on.

DIAGNOSIS AND BREAST LUMPS

REFERRAL TO A SPECIALIST

If you report a lump to your doctor or something shows up on a mammogram, you will be referred to a specialist. Initial tests depend on whether there is a high probability of cancer.

CANCER UNLIKELY

FNAC (see p.127) is used to take a sample of cells from the lump. Laboratory analysis of the aspirated cells will distinguish between a benign lump and a malignant one

CANCER POSSIBLE

If cancer is suspected from your mammogram or because of your age, or if FNAC reveals cancer or is inconclusive, a biopsy is needed to provide a sample of tissue from the lump

BIOPSY

*A cutting-needle biopsy or open biopsy (see p.160) is carried out. If a lump can't be felt, wire localization is used (see **Impalpable lesions**, p.175)*

HISTOLOGY

Histology (analysis of slices of tissue) will diagnose the cancer type and grade the tumor (see p.162)

FURTHER TESTS

Tests are carried out to see if the cancer has spread (see p.161), to determine the outlook for the cancer, and to help plan treatment

Sequence of tests
The tests carried out on a lump determine whether you have cancer and what type, so that you can have the best treatment available.

CUTTING-NEEDLE BIOPSY

1 A special fine-notched needle with a sheath is inserted into the lump.

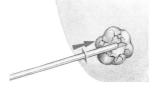

2 The sheath is drawn back, and some tissue from the tumor falls into the notch.

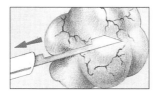

3 The sheath is closed, trapping a tiny core of tumor tissue inside the notch, and the needle is withdrawn.

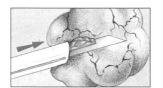

If there is an obvious breast lump the next step is to biopsy it, usually by aspirating the lump (see FNAC, p.127). The sample will be sent to the laboratory for microscopic examination.

CUTTING-NEEDLE BIOPSY

Because FNAC yields only a tiny sample of cells from breast tissue, it's impossible to tell whether they originate from an in situ cancer or an invasive cancer. A cutting-needle biopsy provides a core of cells that can be analysed by a technique known as histology to make this distinction.

Under local anesthetic, a needle not much bigger than that used for FNAC is used to withdraw a fine core of tissue from the lump (see left). The skin is left virtually intact, and there's hardly any discomfort afterward, though there may be a little bruising.

OPEN BIOPSY

This kind of biopsy is an alternative to a cutting-needle biopsy, but as the name implies, the skin is cut open to reveal the lump and remove it with a margin of healthy breast tissue. Any woman over 30 with an obvious breast lump should have it removed, unless she's had a firm diagnosis of cancer from a needle biopsy and can therefore proceed straight to definitive surgical treatment. In practical terms, therefore, open biopsy nearly always means removing the whole lump (lumpectomy, see p.176), and it's usually carried out in the hospital under a local anesthetic, often with intravenous sedation.

Complications of this kind of biopsy are rare – fewer than 1 in 10 cases – but as with any surgical procedure they do occur. The two most likely are a hematoma (bruise) and, less frequently, infection. A hematoma forms from blood oozing into the tissue, and may show as a bruise with a vague lump beneath within a day or two of a biopsy having been done. As with any other bruise, the body simply absorbs the blood and recycles it, and it will disappear after a week or so. Infection, if it occurs, will probably show up within the first week as pain and a raised temperature, and is usually successfully treated with antibiotics. Very rarely a hematoma may become infected and an abscess may form. Antibiotics will be prescribed, and the abscess can be surgically drained (see **Nipple infections**, pp.134–35).

ANALYZING THE BIOPSY

The biopsy or lump is sent to the pathology laboratory where it is very finely sliced, stained to show up cancer cells, and examined under a microscope – a process known as histology. If it is found to be cancerous, a very precise diagnosis of cancer and cancer type can be made. The tumor is also graded (see p.162). At some hospitals specialized tests (see pp.165–66) may be performed on a slice of tumor tissue to reveal features that help to decide treatment and give the patient an idea of future outlook.

An open biopsy is performed purely to remove the lump and send it for analysis. If cancer is found, the surgeon will wait to discuss the treatment options with the woman and her family before any further surgery is carried out. In the past, a biopsy was analyzed instantly while the woman remained under anesthetic, and mastectomy was performed immediately if the lump was cancerous. This was extremely traumatic and is no longer done.

DIAGNOSIS OF SECONDARY SPREAD

In addition to lymph node involvement (see pp.163-64), spread of the disease to the rest of the body is checked by a series of tests generally performed during the initial assessment of anyone with invasive cancer. These include chest X-rays to detect secondaries in the lungs or involvement of the membranes around them (the pleura), X-rays or bone scans of likely sites of bone spread – the skull, spine, pelvis, and hips – and an ultrasound examination to assess the state of the liver. If a woman has no clinical evidence of metastases and her tests are normal, the chances are that she has only local disease. The tests, however, may not reveal microscopic cells. If cancer is suspected but not confirmed, CAT (computerized axial tomography) scans and an MRI (magnetic resonance imaging) may be done. These tests expose a patient to more radiation and are more expensive, so they are performed less routinely.

ONE-STOP DIAGNOSIS

The world's leading cancer centers, such as the Sloan-Kettering Institute in New York and the Royal Marsden Hospital in London, are working toward a 24-hour, one-stop diagnosis for all breast lumps. A woman referred to the center with a lump will be given a diagnostic mammogram or ultrasound scan, depending on her age; FNAC; and, if this is positive or inconclusive, then a cutting-needle biopsy follows. The material for analysis is sent straight to the laboratory, and a firm diagnosis can be made within 24 hours. As well as helping doctors, this service reduces the trauma of waiting for test results.

BREAST BIOFIELD EXAMINATION

Trials are currently under way to establish the effectiveness of a new, non-invasive technique for breast cancer detection. Breast biofield examination (BBE) is based on the fact that there is a tiny electric difference between the interior and exterior of a healthy cell. This is disrupted when the cell becomes cancerous, and the disruption can be detected on the BBE scanner. In its only full trial, on 392 women with suspicious breast lesions, the scanner had a 98 percent accuracy rate, pinpointing 178 of the 182 cancers later detected by biopsy. There are hopes that further successes will mean that BBE will be used more widely in the next two to three years. It could be particularly useful for younger women, in whom mammograms are not very effective.

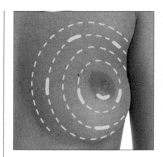

Biopsy incisions
When a biopsy is carried out, the cut is usually made along natural tension lines in the skin to help keep scarring to a minimum.

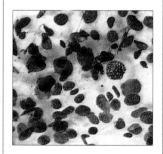

Breast-cancer cells
The cells obtained from a lump by aspiration are stained and examined under a microscope. The dark areas are the cell nuclei. They have stained very heavily and are large, irregular in shape, and divide rapidly.

GRADING, STAGING, AND PROGNOSIS

One of the major aims of doctors is to get a feel for the "virulence" of a cancer. To do this, they use a series of tests to decide on treatment and assess long-term outlook. The tests are intended to determine the aggressiveness of the tumor, and measure how far advanced it is and how far it has spread, if at all, beyond its original site in the breast. The results of such tests will then give an indication of how malignant the cancer is.

GRADING

In one part of the process, cancer cells are examined under the microscope to evaluate their appearance and activity. In breast tissue, the normal cells are identifiable as the kind they are supposed to be. For example, glandular cells form lobules and well-defined ducts. In some cancers, however, the cells have changed so much that it would be difficult to figure out that they arose from breast tissue at all.

The degree of cell differentiation is known as the grade of the tumor and can give a fairly reliable guide to the long-term outlook for the patient. Tumors containing cells that become increasingly unrecognizable as breast tissue are known as "poorly differentiated" or "undifferentiated" and descend through Grades 2 and 3 with a worsening prognosis. Remember, though, that a cell that appears poorly differentiated does not necessarily function poorly.

STAGING OF CANCER

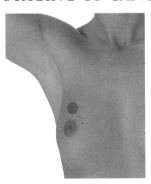

STAGE I
Disease is confined to the breast, with or without dimpling of the skin.

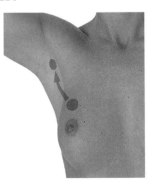

STAGE II
The tumor is larger and the axillary nodes may be affected. Surgery may cure, but some systemic treatment is usually advised.

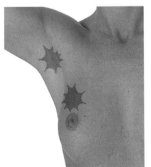

STAGE III
Cancer has invaded the muscles of the chest wall, the overlying skin, or possibly the lymph nodes above the collarbone.

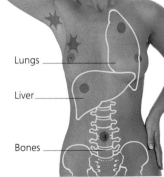

Lungs

Liver

Bones

STAGE IV
The cancer has spread to elsewhere in the body, typically the bones, liver, or lungs.

TUMOR (T)	NODE (N)	METASTASES/SECONDARIES (M)
T1 Tumor less than ¾ inch (2 centimeters) in diameter. (In situ cancers are also staged as T1, whatever their size.)	**N0** Cancer has not spread to the axillary lymph nodes	**M0** No evidence that the cancer has spread to the rest of the body
T2 Tumor ¾–2 inches (2–5 centimeters) in diameter	**N1** Cancer has spread to the axillary lymph nodes on the affected side, but they are still mobile	**M1** Cancer has spread beyond the supraclavicular nodes (above the collarbone)
T3 Tumor greater than 2 inches (5 centimeters) in diameter	**N2** Cancer has spread to the axillary lymph nodes on the affected side, and they have become stuck to one another or to other tissues	
T4 The tumor, whatever its size, has spread to the chest wall or the skin, or the skin is inflamed (inflammatory cancer)	**N3** Internal mammary nodes (behind the breastbone) are involved	

The cells are evaluated according to how many are dividing at once and how rapidly. The more cells that divide simultaneously, the faster the cancer will grow. The rate of division varies as well, and an increase in the speed at which this occurs likewise increases the rate of growth. The blood vessels and lymphatic vessels will also be checked; finding cancer cells there is a sign that the cancer is spreading quickly. All of these examinations of cells are designed to help your doctor make as accurate a prognosis as possible.

STAGING AND THE TNM SYSTEM

Once a breast cancer has been diagnosed and graded, the patient as a whole is staged. The diagram on p.162 sets out the four stages simply. So that every patient can be individually staged, however, the stages can be classified in more detail using the TNM system. It uses a kind of shorthand to describe the size of the tumor (T), whether the lymph nodes are involved (N), and whether there are distant metastases (M) in other parts of the body such as the lungs or liver. The table above explains the scales for each of these.

Size Although size is a fairly crude predictor of the invasive potential of the tumor, the larger the tumor, the more likely it is to have had time to spread to the axillary lymph nodes. Even small tumors may have spread, however. Most women whose tumors measure less than ½ inch (1 centimeter) and whose lymph nodes are free of disease have an excellent prognosis.

Nodal status In terms of assessing a patient's future outlook, the crucial factor against which all others should be weighed is spread to the axillary lymph nodes; the more nodes in the armpit that are involved, the worse the prognosis. With a node-negative cancer, 7 women out of 10 will be alive 10 years later;

The TNM system
Three factors are taken into acount when staging cancer: the size of the tumor, whether it has spread to the axillary lymph nodes, and whether there are metastases elsewhere in the body.

with a node-positive cancer, only 5 or fewer out of 10. Adjuvant chemotherapy (see pp.187–88) is now routinely given to premenopausal women with involved nodes. Most other women, whether their nodes are free of cancer or not, would benefit from adjuvant systemic therapy, usually tamoxifen.

Metastasis The presence of secondary tumors elsewhere in the body can be detected by special tests (see p.161). If the lymph nodes above the collarbone (the supraclavicular nodes) are involved, these are regarded as metastases. Distant metastases in the lungs, liver, or bones automatically put the cancer at Stage IV, so their presence is a very serious sign.

PLANNING TREATMENT

The staging system was designed by doctors for two purposes: first as a basis for deciding on the most appropriate treatment, and second to be able to give you an idea of future outlook.

Once you have been staged, decisions about treatment can be made. You have the right to discuss all possible alternatives so that you and your family participate in all decisions. One tool that is often found useful in trying to understand the "personality" of a cancer is to compare it to a dog. Depending on the stage or prognostic factors, the cancer can be placed on a scale that ranges from a "poodle" to a "rottweiler." This type of association can then help you and your relatives to visualize the disease and get a feel for it – it obviously works, as many patients ask if theirs was a "rottweiler" when the results are being discussed. You can also be helped to come to terms with the diagnosis by being given a tape recording of the "bad news consultation" to take home, so ask for one, and by having a friend or relative with you for moral support when the news is broken.

SURVIVAL

There is so much about any cancer that can never be known that, although many women who get breast cancer do not die of it, doctors would still be reluctant to say that those women had been cured. We still do not have reliable tests to tell us exactly where a cancer has spread to, and we are still not very good at predicting those that will, so we prefer to talk about survival. Usually we measure five-year and ten-year survival rates, and express them as a percentage. If you are told by your doctor that your cancer has a five-year survival rate of 80 percent, it means that, of 10 women with your disease, with a tumor of the same grade and stage, and of the same degree of aggressiveness, 8 could expect to be alive in five years' time.

PROGNOSIS AND OUTLOOK

As well as the known factors, there are probably many unknown ones that affect the outcome of breast cancer, and even after a very careful assessment it may still be difficult for your doctor to give you a precise outlook. Breast cancer can defy all predictions. Some women who have widespread disease, and who, on the face of it, appear to have an utterly hopeless prognosis, may then go on to live to a ripe old age. At the other end of the scale, those with small tumors diagnosed at an early stage and treated very aggressively with potentially curative surgery and adjuvant therapy have only a 7 out of 10 cure rate. The stage of the tumor is crucial in assessing five-year survival rate for breast cancer: the five-year survival rate of 85 percent for Stage I tumor sufferers falls to less than 10 percent for those with Stage IV tumors.

About 1 in 3 women who are treated vigorously for early breast cancer will then have a normal life expectation. Of the remainder, those who get local recurrence can often be treated adequately with radiotherapy. The sad fact is that only about half of the women who see breast-cancer surgeons see them early enough, when the disease is eminently treatable and curable; the other half leave it too long before seeking help.

On the whole, however, the news is good. Most women with breast cancer still have a reasonable expectation of life by comparison with cancers of the lung, stomach, or ovary, where the outlook is much more dire. Many women can expect to live in comfort for many years after treatment, even if their disease cannot be classed as cured. As breast cancer is mainly a disease of older women, many will die from other causes or simply from old age rather than from their breast tumor.

PROGNOSTIC INDEX

Doctors strive to come up with simple mathematical calculations in order to give their patients a view of future survival. For example, here is one index; it was developed by the breast research group in Nottingham, England. Based on an analysis of many hundreds of cases of breast cancer where survival and time to relapse were carefully measured, it's called the Nottingham Prognostic Index (NPI), and it combines the size of the tumor, the grade of the tumor, and the stage of the axillary lymph nodes in the following way:

NPI = (0.2 × tumor size in centimeters) + grade + stage

For example, a Stage I tumor 1 centimeter across with Grade 1 cells would have an NPI of (0.2 × 1) + 1 + 1, giving a total of 2.2. The lower the NPI, the better the prognosis.

SPECIAL RESEARCH TESTS

Over the years, researchers have attempted to develop special tests that will give us an even better idea of the aggressiveness of breast tumors, future outlook, and survival. These markers, as they are called, require very advanced technology and are by no means performed at all centers. They are confined to units carrying out advanced research programs and are not therefore generally available. Much work is going on in the science of markers, because they may help us to predict the future.

Although most of these tests are of research interest only, it's hoped that their future use will help identify groups of patients who would do better with one kind of treatment or another. A few breast cancers do not fall into clear treatment groups, and special tests to find out their nature could be helpful.

Using these predictors of outcome, it's sometimes possible to define a subgroup of node-negative women whose outlook is so good that no adjuvant treatment is needed after surgery. In research units where these special tests are available, they can provide useful information.

Estrogen receptors (ERs) Estrogen receptors were the first of the biological markers to be studied; approximately 60 percent of cancers contain detectable ERs. A tumor that has ERs is sensitive to estrogen and has a slightly better prognosis than one that doesn't. There is less than a 10 percent difference in survival rate between patients with ER-positive tumors and those whose tumors are ER-negative. ER-positive patients live longer, however, and tend to respond better to hormones and chemotherapy after relapse.

Epidermal growth-factor receptor (EGFr) All cells have receptors that are "switched on" by growth factors telling the cell to multiply. In altered cells, the receptors don't wait to be told what to do, but cause the cells to multiply uncontrollably. About half of breast-cancer cases have altered receptors. Tumors that are EGFr-negative generally have a better outlook for recovery than those that are positive.

EGFr tends to correspond to other factors that indicate a poor outlook, such as a high tumor grade. It is also correlated with a shorter survival time and a short time to relapse. EGFr gives some indication of the likely response to endocrine therapy, because patients without EGFr respond better. Elderly patients treated with tamoxifen alone are five times more likely to respond if their tumors are EGFr-negative.

Ki-67 In simple terms, this measures the speed of cell growth and division. Generally speaking, the faster the cells are dividing, the more aggressive the tumor. This in turn means that the spread of the cancer throughout the body is likely to occur earlier and be faster. The chance of metastases is high and the outlook poorer than with slower cell changes.

erbB-2 Research has shown that women who relapse have extra copies of the altered form of this gene, and higher levels of the protein it produces. The more *erbB-2* present, the poorer the prognosis seems to be. Even when other prognostic factors like stage and grade are taken into account, those tumors that are *erbB-2* positive have a worse outcome. This is important in deciding treatment, because it can indicate that the outlook is poor even where other indicators might be more positive.

Cathepsin D Patients with low levels of the enzyme cathepsin D and positive axillary nodes invariably outlive those with high levels of cathepsin D and negative nodes. It is therefore quite a powerful predictor of outcome.

p53 This is a gene mutation (see p.142) that is known to be present in about half of all breast cancers. An abnormality of *p53* gives an increased risk of ovarian and bowel cancer as well as breast cancer. When the gene is normal it restricts cell growth; when it is damaged, cells are able to grow out of control. It is hoped that research will produce a drug that would counteract the effects of the damaged gene.

ON FINDING A LUMP

So much media attention is given to breast cancer nowadays that it would be difficult for any woman to ignore the potential significance of a breast lump. The sad fact is that on finding a lump, almost all women underestimate the chances of survival and overestimate the chances of dying. Finding a breast lump is therefore a shocking experience for everyone.

DENIAL

One of the most common coping strategies for us all is denial, a natural protective mechanism that helps us to go on in times of stress or shock. Where cancer is involved, however, such delay in reporting symptoms will worsen the outlook for the disease. You may try to convince yourself that a lump is nothing to worry about until it can no longer be ignored. By then the tumor is difficult to treat and the chances of survival are low. Recent studies have given us a clear picture of the characteristics and personality types of the women most likely to delay reporting a breast lump:

• older women

• women of lower social class or little education

• depressed or anxious personalities or those who habitually resort to denial in a crisis

• women who are very fearful of cancer and of surgery and don't believe they can be helped or cured

• women who are inhibited about their bodies.

Paradoxically, knowledge as opposed to ignorance about breast cancer may inhibit some women from seeking advice at the proper time; one study showed that female health-care professionals, especially nurses, tended to report their lumps later and generally had larger tumors than other women.

THE IMPLICATIONS OF DELAY

Finding a lump in the breast is always scary, but don't become so frightened that you don't seek help immediately. It's been estimated that approximately 1 in 5 women with symptoms of breast cancer delays seeking advice for three months or more, and some research has suggested that this delay could well be contributing to the high mortality rates in Great Britain.

The interval between finding a breast lump and having a diagnosis confirmed is the most stressful part of finding a lump in your breast. A group of women who were studied before and after having their lump diagnosed as benign were found to suffer severe impairment of critical thinking and concentration together with profound anxiety before the diagnosis. Fewer than 1 in 8 women gives breast loss as her primary concern; nearly 6 out of 10 are more distressed at the prospect of having cancer.

I told myself that I was being silly, that it just couldn't be cancer and the lump would go away, but underneath I was terrified. I didn't mention it to my husband for weeks because there never seemed to be a good time. If he seemed happy, I didn't want to spoil it, and if he seemed down I didn't want to worry him. Finally I mentioned it to my sister. She said I should go straight to the doctor, and she came with me.

LIZ, 56, MARKETING MANAGER

ON HEARING THE DIAGNOSIS

Individual coping strategies and personality factors will affect your response to the news that you have breast cancer. Social support can help you, and the communications skills of your medical carers, especially the surgeon who breaks the news, are very important. Your reaction may have several stages; denial, fighting back, brave acceptance, depressed acceptance, and a mixture of helplessness and hopelessness are all possible.

Most of us are likely to go through stages of depressed acceptance, where we acknowledge that we have a potentially fatal disease but are overwhelmed with fears for ourselves and our families. At worst, we may feel that there is no hope for us; however much we have to live for, we may not be able to muster the energy to fight for it.

SUPPORT

Those of us who have supportive family and friends are more able to cope with this kind of life crisis. Hearing the bad news in the presence of a close relative or friend reduces anxiety and depression for a long time afterward, and he or she will probably remember more clearly than you what the doctor said. The presence of a trusted ally, be it spouse, partner, friend, or relative, is useful in the long term to help you accept that you have cancer.

THE FAMILY

The needs of your family are sometimes overlooked. It's easy to assume that they will be able to keep their feelings in check and be ready to offer support. Families do, however, suffer along with you and very often reflect your mood. One study showed that if a patient with cancer is depressed or anxious there is a very high probability that the next of kin will be also.

Partners Your partner is likely to feel responsible for helping you to adjust successfully to your disease and to your new body after the operation. He may suffer considerable emotional distress but pretend to hide this behind a confident pose, assuming that this will help you. Unfortunately this attitude may lead to misunderstandings. You may feel that your partner is not being sensitive to your feelings and doesn't realize the seriousness of the situation or can't share your fears. It is natural when a loved one is in distress to try to offer advice, be cheery, or somehow "sort things out," but this may not be what you need: more often you just want someone to listen and understand.

Relationships are always affected in some way by a woman's diagnosis of breast cancer; with fragile relationships this burden may prove to be the final straw. For the majority of women, however, it's a time when the commitment, love, and affection of her family and friends are reaffirmed.

At the time of the diagnosis, good information and counseling should be provided to the person closest to you, as this "significant other" will be a crucial factor in your long-term adjustment. In the end, most couples feel their relationships to be at least the same, sometimes even better.

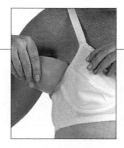

CHAPTER NINE

TREATING BREAST CANCER

The detection and diagnosis of breast cancer is only the first step in combating the disease. All women should know what treatment options are open to them, the techniques involved, and the support they are entitled to receive, especially when coming to terms with life after treatment.

TREATMENT OPTIONS

If you are diagnosed as having breast cancer, it's very important that you should be fully aware of the various treatment options that are open to you. Twenty years ago, radical mastectomies were the rule; today, surgery aims to conserve the breast if at all possible. At the same time, highly sophisticated reconstructive surgery has been developed so that a woman who loses her breast has the option of replacing it. Advanced techniques for calculating future risks mean that we can place a woman in a very clearly defined group and choose a tailor-made treatment program specially for her, giving her the best possible chance of a cure.

BREAST CENTERS

Women with breast cancer are increasingly treated at specialized centers, such as those at the Sloan-Kettering Institute, New York, and Guy's Hospital, London. These centers offer women the best possible care, and ensure close co-operation between an interested and sympathetic oncologist, surgeon, pathologist, radiologist, and radiotherapist, which allows rapid and accurate diagnosis and appropriate treatment. The team will also include counselors or special breast-care nurses (see p.171) trained to deal with the emotional and psychological aspects of breast cancer. Specialized breast cancer centers also supervise adjuvant therapy such as radiotherapy, chemotherapy, and hormone therapy – and breast reconstruction if desired – so all your treatments are kept under one roof with a minimum of travel and disturbance during follow-up.

CONSERVING THE BREAST

Women who develop breast cancer are in a much more fortunate position now than in the past; many more treatment options are open to you, and preserving the breast need pose no hazard to life. Not so long ago it was thought that mastectomy, including the removal of all the lymph nodes in the armpit, was necessary in every case to give a woman the best chance of survival. This is no longer true. Doctors have abandoned the idea that this kind of extensive surgery should be routine, and without sacrificing results have greatly improved recovery after surgery. With conservative treatment, the worst complication of breast surgery, swelling of the arm (lymphedema, see p.194), is now rare.

Surgeons nowadays believe in conserving the breast whenever possible or choosing the least extensive operation that is appropriate. With early breast cancer, lumpectomy is nearly always an option. This means that very small tumors can be dealt with, leaving the breast virtually intact.

The choice of operation is based only partly on medical grounds. Because the many different approaches to treatment all offer about the same success rate, there is nothing to prevent your preferences from carrying weight. The outlook for the disease is affected more by the tumor's stage and grade (see pp.162–63) when it is diagnosed than by the type of surgery performed.

Any choice should be made in consultation with you and your family. Not all patients are suitable for breast conservation, however, and you would be well advised to listen to your doctors when a more radical approach is advocated. If lumpectomy is attempted in inappropriate cases – on a large tumor, for example – the cosmetic results and disease control can be poor.

THE LOSS OF A BREAST

Whenever the subject of mastectomy is discussed, make sure that you and your family understand precisely the extent of the operation. Ask to see some photographs of women after mastectomy – this will give you an idea of how your body will look after surgery. You'll almost certainly need time and space and counseling to get used to the idea of a different-looking body that at first may seem alien to you.

You will have much greater difficulty coming to terms with your new appearance than your partner, family, and friends will. They are far more concerned about your well-being and long-term health than about your body's appearance. It's understandable, however, that you are not. A woman's self-image is often indistinguishable from her self-esteem. Fortunately, doctors and surgeons now understand this and should be willing to give you all the help you require along the way.

You are entitled to have a cosmetically acceptable result after surgery and be pleased with your appearance when dressed, even in low necklines. This can be achieved by the use of false breasts (see p.195). Reconstructive surgery (see p.189) is also widely available to restore both breast contour and a nipple if you so wish. Don't be afraid to ask your surgeon about these things or worry that you will be thought vain or frivolous for being concerned about your appearance. You have the right to expect your surgeon to be sympathetic to these concerns, and most surgeons are.

BREAST CANCER: YOUR BILL OF RIGHTS

• A prompt referral by your general practitioner to a team specializing in the diagnosis and treatment of breast cancer, including a consultant
• A firm diagnosis within one week
• The opportunity of a confirmed diagnosis before consenting to treatment, including surgery
• Access to a special breast-care nurse trained to give information and psychological support
• Full information about types of surgery (including breast reconstruction where appropriate) and the role of adjuvant medical treatments such as radiotherapy, chemotherapy, hormone therapy including tamoxifen, and so on

• A clear and detailed explanation of the aims of the proposed treatments and their benefits and any possible side effects
• As much time as you need to consider your treatment options and gather information
• A sensitive and complete breast prosthesis service, where appropriate
• The opportunity to meet a former breast-cancer patient who has been trained to offer support
• Information on all support services available to breast-cancer patients and their families

ASSESSING TREATMENTS: CLINICAL TRIALS

Although many attempts have been made to compare the survival rates after different operations, meaningful comparisons have always been difficult. One of the major hurdles has been to perform a study that would compare survival rates with mastectomy against more conservative surgery. Differences between the success rates of operations are small, and to reveal any truly significant margins tens of thousands of women had to be studied for many years. In addition, the outcome of the different surgical procedures is influenced by adjuvant therapies such as hormonal therapy, chemotherapy, and radiotherapy.

The acid test of success for any new procedure is its ability to help women with breast cancer, and this can be ascertained only from clinical trials; these trials give the information on which treatment for breast cancer can be based.

This raises the question of whether it is really justifiable to ask a woman to undergo a particular treatment that may not have the same success as others. It helps to bear in mind that all new treatments are carefully researched in preliminary studies, and that a full clinical trial will be carried out only if this initial research clearly suggests that the new treatment may be better than the current standard treatment. Any woman who takes part in a clinical trial is free to withdraw at any stage and be given standard treatment instead.

CONDUCTING TRIALS

In order to remove uncertainties and variation from the results of trials, it is necessary to perform what is called a "randomized double-blind" test. "Randomized" means that women taking part are assigned by chance to either the standard treatment or the tested one. "Double-blind" means that neither the researcher nor the woman knows to which treatment she's been assigned. This information is kept secret until the results have been collated. These arrangements aim for an impartial result; if a researcher doesn't know what treatment is being given, his or her preconceptions won't affect the results.

Because women are given treatments randomly, they must be fully informed about the implications of the trial before they give their informed consent to participate. This requires a degree of selflessness and altruism and raises a possible worry that such women may not constitute a representative sample.

Clinical trials are expensive to run and require a lot of time and effort, so many clinicians find it difficult to undertake them. In addition, many doctors feel a moral dilemma about pursuing a woman's informed consent because of the apparent element of coercion. On the plus side, it's evident that patients who take part in clinical trials receive marginally better treatment and do better than those who don't, possibly because they are monitored so closely. Yet fewer than 2 percent of eligible patients ever enter a clinical trial. One suggestion aimed at increasing such participation is that teams of women "proselytizers" who have taken part in trials themselves might be trained to offer information and counseling to eligible women. Given the importance of these trials in improving the treatment of breast cancer, it is vital that women are encouraged to take part.

THE APPROACH TO BREAST-CANCER TREATMENT

When your doctors consider the treatment of a breast cancer they are taking into consideration several different factors that will influence treatment and long-term outlook. Doctors have to tread a narrow line between the most effective treatment for your condition and the need to cause you the least trauma, both physical and mental. This balance is not always easy to achieve and requires your full and frank input and cooperation. In addition, the better informed you are about the issues involved, the more active a part you can take in deciding your own treatment. This will not only help your doctor and surgeon in their task but may also give you added strength in fighting your cancer. The first thing you need to understand is that treatment of breast cancer falls into three distinct areas:

• treatment of the lump, usually with surgery

• treatment of the lymph nodes in the axilla, with surgical clearance as a rule

• adjuvant therapy where appropriate, which could be radiotherapy to clear any remaining cancer cells from the breast after surgery, or chemotherapy or hormone therapy to catch any spread of the cancer to the rest of the body

Surgery and radiotherapy are referred to as local treatments because they treat only the area where the tumor has occurred. Chemotherapy and hormone therapy are called systemic treatments because they treat the whole body.

The state-of-the-art treatment for breast cancer appears to be that pioneered by Guy's Hospital, London, and centers in Paris, Milan, and Boston. The first step is exact diagnosis with cutting-needle biopsy (see p.160); a short while later (three to seven days), after you've been fully consulted, a single operation will remove the lump and clear the axillary lymph nodes. Precise radiotherapy to the tumor site is given, which avoids excessive irradiation of the skin and deeper organs. This gives results at least as good as mastectomy, with much less heartache. Nearly every woman is considered for some form of systemic adjuvant treatment (see p.185). If you have a tumor less than 1 centimeter in diameter and you're node-negative (see p.163), you belong to the only group of women for whom systemic adjuvant therapy is not considered necessary.

PLANNING TREATMENT

Breast cancer is usually referred to as either early or advanced; this reflects whether the cancer is operable or not. "Early" usually encompasses Stages I and II (see p.162), and "advanced," Stages III and IV. These terms are also used to reflect the aggressiveness of the tumor – some patients do quite well with large ulcerated cancers that have been present for some time but that are clearly not rapidly growing because they have not spread to other parts of the body. A small primary tumor, on the other hand, can spread quickly to other organs if it is very aggressive. The treatment given in cases of early breast cancer – that is, cancer that has not yet spread beyond the axillary lymph nodes – has three main aims:

• to control the disease locally – that is, at the site of the tumor – and prevent local recurrence

• to treat any micrometastatic disease (tiny, undetectable secondary spread) so as to increase the chances of survival

• to conserve as much of the breast as possible and be minimally disfiguring.

Local control is of prime importance and, as proven at Guy's Hospital, can largely be achieved by removal of the lump with a margin of healthy breast tissue, followed by a course of radiotherapy in some form. If you have a large or aggressive tumor, you'll be asked to consider mastectomy. All but patients with very early cancer will be given adjuvant therapy in some form; for nearly all older women this is the drug tamoxifen (see p.186).

If a tumor is allowed to reach an advanced state, then the likelihood of metastases is much greater. For this reason local treatment alone is deemed inadequate and systemic treatment is the rule. The most common systemic treatment for premenopausal women is chemotherapy, which works on cancer throughout the body and may shrink your tumor to an operable size.

PRIMARY MEDICAL THERAPY

Research at the excellent Milan breast center in Italy showed that chemotherapy *before* the operation can reduce four out of five large tumors to under 3 centimeters, allowing them to be treated with more conservative surgery and reducing physical and emotional trauma. Tumors have been clearly seen to shrink and disappear on successive mammograms, although microcalcification may remain. Wherever it is practiced, primary medical treatment is always followed by additional surgical treatment to avoid the chance of local relapse.

BREAST CANCER IN PREGNANCY

It seems that breast cancer is no more likely to arise in pregnancy and behaves no differently during pregnancy than at any other time. Be assured that the hormonal changes of pregnancy, when levels of estrogen are high, do not seem to make the situation worse.

Treatment depends on how advanced the pregnancy is. Radiotherapy is not considered an option. Toxic anticancer drugs are not given in the first three months, since they do affect the developing fetus; if chemotherapy is the treatment of choice during the first trimester, the doctor may suggest an abortion. In the US, a mastectomy is the standard treatment for pregnant women with breast cancer. For many, a lumpectomy would be preferable, but it is usually followed by radiotherapy to the breast (see p.183), which could affect the fetus. If a woman is due within eight weeks and radiotherapy is recommended, treatment may be postponed until after delivery.

SURGERY

In most cases local conservative therapy will be achieved with surgery. It is time-consuming to treat small tumors with chemotherapy and radiotherapy; large tumors need large doses of radiation which can distort and disfigure breast tissue. Treatment should be effective and result in an acceptable-looking breast; in this regard the ratio of breast size to tumor size is decisive.

Lumpectomy is the most common primary treatment for smaller breast cancers and can generally be relied on to give a good cosmetic result (see p.177). If yours is a large tumor in the center of the breast or one with several different areas of focus, a mastectomy may be preferable. A lumpectomy in such cases may not be cosmetically attractive, and it may be impossible to provide a satisfactory prosthesis for a very distorted breast. A reconstruction operation is always an option either during the initial surgery or later. Chemotherapy or hormone therapy prior to surgery may be offered if you have a large tumor, to reduce its size and allow a smaller area of breast tissue to be removed.

IMPALPABLE LESIONS

Lesions that can't be felt by self-examination or by your doctor but show up on mammography as shadows with tiny white dots of calcification can be accurately located with mammographic guidance. Small, solid tumors can also be localized with the use of ultrasound. A small wire is inserted into the center of the tumor and left in place to indicate the tumor's position. The surgeon dissects down onto the wire so that the whole of the tumor can be cut out, leaving no remnants. A block of tissue 1–2 centimeters around the lesion is excised (removed). This is then X-rayed while the patient is still asleep to confirm that the mammographic abnormality has been completely excised. This technique makes it possible to achieve complete excision in almost 100 percent of impalpable cancers.

LOCATING THE LESION
Using an ultrasound image as a guide, the radiologist inserts a fine wire into the lesion. The wire is then fixed in place and left there to guide the surgeon to the lesion.

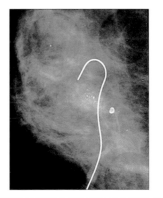

LOCALIZATION WIRE
This mammogram shows the wire in position in the breast just before surgery. The cluster of white dots that are visible inside the hook of the wire are distinct microcalcifications (see p.66).

Mastectomy is major surgery, and you deserve to have an expert surgeon. It is recommended that women with breast cancer be treated by only those doctors who see more than 30 new cancers a year, who can offer a full range of treatment options, and who work within a team of specialists.

CONSERVATIVE THERAPY

Breast conservation is most suitable if your lump is less than 4 centimeters in diameter felt on clinical examination or shown on a mammogram. Minimal nodal involvement with no distant metastases is a requirement. The TNM system (see p.163) classes such a tumor as T1 or T2, N0 or N1, and M0.

If you have large breasts and a tumor bigger than 4 centimeters you might also be suitable. There is no age limit. If you are elderly, provided you are fit, you should be treated in exactly the same way as younger patients.

Breast conservation will not be offered if it would result in an unacceptable cosmetic result. This would normally include the majority of cancers in the center of the breast and those that are over 4 centimeters in diameter.

Women with more than one focus of cancer have a high local recurrence rate with breast conservation and are better treated with mastectomy, ideally with immediate breast reconstruction. Cancer in both breasts can be treated by a bilateral conservation, but you may prefer bilateral mastectomy, again with immediate reconstruction.

Overview of surgery
Any cancerous tumor will have to be removed, but the extent of the surgery will depend on the size of the tumor, its position, whether it forms a discrete lump, and how aggressive it seems to be. Surgery to the axilla will be carried out at the same time.

OPERATION	WHEN SUITABLE	WHAT'S REMOVED	TYPE OF OPERATION
Lumpectomy	*Small tumor (under 4 cm), not central, not aggressive, no evidence of spread. Larger tumor (more than 4 cm) in large breasts*	*Lump and, in most cases, 1 cm of healthy breast tissue all around. Rest of breast left intact*	*Fairly minor operation under local anesthetic. One day in the hospital*
Partial mastectomy (e.g., quadrantectomy)	*Small tumor with ill-defined edge*	*Lump and some of the surrounding tissue. The amount will vary according to the size and position of the lump*	*Fairly minor operation under general anesthetic. One day in the hospital*
Simple or total mastectomy	*Multicentric DCIS (see p.156) or extensive DCIS*	*Removes all of the breast including the axillary tail (the part of the breast that pierces the muscles of the chest wall), nipple, areola, and surrounding skin*	*Major operation under general anesthetic. One to two days in the hospital*
Modified radical mastectomy	*Aggressive tumors over 4 cm in diameter*	*As for simple mastectomy, but the pectoralis minor muscle is also removed*	*Major operation under general anesthetic. One to two days in the hospital, longer if reconstruction required*

LUMPECTOMY

Wherever possible, lumpectomy is now the treatment of choice for breast cancer, for its cosmetic qualities and because it's less emotionally traumatic. As long as the postoperative dose of radiotherapy is sufficiently high, only the lump itself need be removed, but most surgeons still go for the safety margin of 1 centimeter of normal breast tissue around it. The minimum amount of skin is removed to give the best cosmetic result. When a large amount of skin needs to be excised – if the lump is very near the surface, for example – the cosmetic results are likely to be rather poor, and your doctor should make you aware of this. Most surgeons remove the lymph nodes from the armpit at the same time. The operation itself is a fairly minor procedure carried out under local anesthetic. Many patients are able to return to work the next day, and soreness disappears within seven to ten days.

MASTECTOMY

In the past, mastectomy was the treatment of choice for breast cancer, as it was thought that the tumor spread by growing outward from the primary growth in the center. It therefore seemed logical to perform ever more extensive surgery to attempt to get beyond the growing edge of the tumor. Radical surgery is no longer the norm for breast cancer, and there are currently several possible variations of mastectomy.

TREATMENT OF AXILLA	ADJUVANT THERAPY	COSMETIC RESULTS	COMPLICATIONS
Axillary nodes removed except with DCIS. Occasionally radiotherapy, or no treatment may be recommended instead	Radiotherapy to rest of breast. If nodes are involved, chemotherapy or tamoxifen is recommended according to age (see p.186)	Good if lump small. Breastfeeding still possible	Rarely bruising
Axillary lymph nodes are sampled or cleared and the tumor staged	Local radiotherapy to the breast. Chemotherapy or tamoxifen	There may be a large dent in the breast, depending on how much tissue is removed	Rarely bruising
Lymph nodes and patient's estrogen receptor status may be sampled and the tumor staged (see p.163).	With DCIS, chemotherapy or tamoxifen generally not recommended	The chest is flat with a horizontal scar. Can wear low-necked clothes with a prosthesis (see p.194). A breast mound and false nipple can be fashioned surgically later (see p.189)	Bruising and discomfort, possibly stiff shoulder
All nodes can be easily cleared out	Possibly hormones, chemotherapy, or tamoxifen	Flat chest with horizontal scar. Can wear low-necked clothes with prosthesis. A breast mound and false nipple can be surgically fashioned later	Bruising and discomfort, possibly stiff shoulder. Very rarely lymphedema of the arm (see p.194)

• A partial mastectomy, as its name implies, involves removing part of the breast. (Segmental excision and quadrantectomy are versions of this type of operation and remove varying amounts of tissue.) A sample of the axillary nodes will be taken at the same time or they may be cleared. The operation can leave a misshapen breast, depending on how much tissue is removed. Knowing this, women often opt for a total mastectomy.

• A simple or total mastectomy removes all the breast tissue including the nipple and areola and the axillary tail. Some or all of the axillary lymph nodes may be removed at the same time.

• Modified radical mastectomy is a total mastectomy and may include removal of the pectoralis minor muscle to facilitate full axillary clearance. It is the favored operation of many breast centers where lumpectomy is not feasible.

BREAST SURGERY

There are several possible operations, and doctors will aim to remove the minimum amount of tissue necessary to get rid of the cancer. The extent of surgery is determined by the size and position of the tumor, whether the lump has a well-defined outline, how aggressive it appears to be, and whether the cancer has spread.

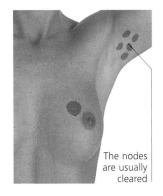

The nodes are usually cleared

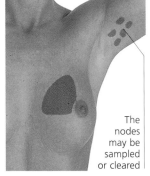

The nodes may be sampled or cleared

PARTIAL MASTECTOMY
Where the cancer doesn't have a distinct outline, the lump is removed with a larger amount of the surrounding tissue than for a lumpectomy (a quadrantectomy, for example). The axillary lymph nodes are also sampled or cleared.

LUMPECTOMY
The lump is removed with a ½-inch (1-centimeter) margin of healthy tissue to give the best cosmetic result. The axillary nodes are usually removed too.

SIMPLE OR TOTAL MASTECTOMY
All of the breast tissue is removed, including the nipple and areola and the axillary tail. No muscles are removed. The axillary lymph nodes may be sampled or cleared.

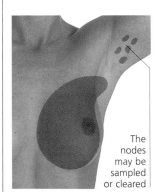

The nodes may be sampled or cleared

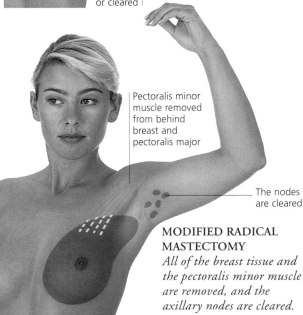

Pectoralis minor muscle removed from behind breast and pectoralis major

The nodes are cleared

MODIFIED RADICAL MASTECTOMY
All of the breast tissue and the pectoralis minor muscle are removed, and the axillary nodes are cleared.

• In radical mastectomy the pectoralis major muscle is also removed if the tumor is extensive and involves the muscle. Radical mastectomies were once standard, but the availability of adjuvant therapy has rendered them largely unnecessary.

Mastectomy is a major operation and you'll have to stay in the hospital for four to eight days, depending on the type of surgery performed. If your shoulder is stiff afterward you can do exercises to get it back to normal (see pp.196–97).

TIMING THE OPERATION

Although studies at Guy's Hospital, London, and later in Milan, Italy, and at the Sloan-Kettering Institute in New York suggest that premenopausal women who have breast surgery during the second half of the menstrual cycle – the so-called luteal phase – have improved survival, most literature does not support this conclusion. Progesterone, which increases during the luteal phase, is thought to be influential. However, rather than the increased progesterone, it may be the presence, in some women, of progesterone receptors on the cancer cells that accounts for the better outcomes.

A WORD ABOUT MASTECTOMY

More than 80 percent of breast cancers are caught early enough to be suitable for lumpectomy, yet the American College of Surgeons says that only 35 percent are so treated. In New York, hospitals just miles apart have widely varying lumpectomy rates. Why? In Colorado, where three-quarters of women get mastectomies, studies show that it's doctors who are responsible for such low lumpectomy rates, advocating mastectomies even though we've had scientific evidence since 1989 to show that lumpectomy plus radiation is just as good as mastectomy. According to some professors in the US this is because surgeons have not been keeping up with the medical literature. This is sad, because a study has revealed that half of mastectomy patients, when asked, said they'd choose lumpectomy if they could make the decision again.

In 1992, a report in the *New England Journal of Medicine* showed that teaching hospitals, where surgeons tend to be more up to date, have a higher lumpectomy rate. And women who have lumpectomies return to everyday life more quickly and report better sex lives. You have the right to a lumpectomy if you're eligible, but you may have to change surgeons to get one.

Approaches to surgery
This table shows the wide variation between the proportion of lumpectomies and mastectomies in regions of the US. Such variations can occur in any country, and show that women are not always being offered the most appropriate treatment.

REGION	MASTECTOMY	LUMPECTOMY	OTHER
Northeast	43.4%	46.9%	9.7%
Midwest	54.0%	35.1%	10.9%
South	63.6%	24.8%	11.6%
Southwest	69.2%	22.9%	7.9%
West	56.2%	39.3%	4.5%

TREATING THE AXILLA

A lymph node infiltrated by cancer has ceased to perform any useful service to your body. Furthermore, cancer can only spread further. Affected axillary lymph nodes must therefore be removed or treated vigorously. The treatment of axillary lymph nodes is still debated by surgeons and radiotherapists. The surgical options range from sampling – that is, removing a limited number of nodes (with or without subsequent radiotherapy) – to complete surgical clearance of the axillary nodes. There are some radiotherapists who would advocate radiotherapy as the first and only treatment. The consensus among most specialists, however, is that complete axillary node clearance should be the first step wherever possible.

All doctors treating breast cancer are concerned to know the status of the axillary nodes because it remains the single best predictor of long-term survival. Added to this, some of the most important treatment choices and decisions are based on axillary node status. In order to get a true idea of the axillary node status, some form of surgical sampling is needed, because as yet there are no good imaging techniques for the axilla. The role of axillary surgery is therefore twofold: to stage the tumor and to treat axillary disease. Radiotherapy may treat the axilla well enough, but it precludes staging of the tumor – information that most oncologists consider crucial.

Logically, then, surgery is superior to radiotherapy, and many surgeons feel that if they are going to operate on the axilla, complete clearance of the lymph nodes gives a better outlook than just sampling.

STAGING THE AXILLA

The most accurate way to stage the axilla is to examine the lymph nodes starting with the shallowest and working through progressively deeper levels. We speak of three levels, I being the shallowest and III the deepest. On average there are 14 lymph nodes at Level I, five at Level II, and two at Level III. When there is no Level I involvement in the cancer, the likelihood of disease at Levels II and III is very slight.

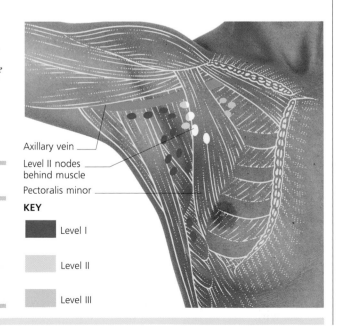

Axillary vein
Level II nodes behind muscle
Pectoralis minor

KEY

- Level I
- Level II
- Level III

HOW LEVEL I NODES PREDICT YOUR CHANCES

Number of nodes positive at Level I	1	2	3	4	5
Chances of positive nodes at Levels II & III	12%	19%	37%	40%	84%

From the point of view of deciding on systemic therapy, sampling the axillary nodes is more important in premenopausal than postmenopausal women; this is because for postmenopausal women tamoxifen is usually the treatment of choice, regardless of whether they are node-positive or node-negative (see p.186).

DETERMINING SPREAD

Sampling of nodes at Level I (see below) can be a good indication of how far the tumor has spread. Surgical options include single-node biopsy, removing a sample of four nodes, Level I clearance, Level II clearance, and Level III clearance. Where surgery is preferred to radiotherapy, complete clearance rather than sampling is necessary. Even a single positive node at Level I may be a sign of involvement at Levels II and III. To be sure that there is no involvement at the deeper levels, however, we need a large sample of clear nodes. Research studies performed in Europe have shown that at least 10 lymph nodes at Level I have to be sampled in order to give 90 percent confidence in predicting that there is no lymphatic spread of the breast tumor.

There is a direct relationship between the size of your tumor and whether it has already spread to the axillary lymph nodes. If your tumor was detected by screening, however, it's less likely to have axillary spread than if you'd found it yourself, regardless of its size. For this reason it has become standard practice in many breast centers for patients with breast cancer to have axillary node samples taken at Levels I and II as a first step. The extent of the sample varies according to a variety of factors, which should be discussed thoroughly and individually with the surgeon.

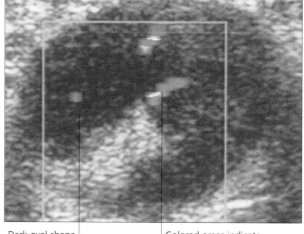

Dark oval shape is lymph node

Colored areas indicate strong blood flow

Cancerous lymph node
This ultrasound image shows a lymph node that has been infiltrated by cancer. The dark oval shape is the node. The large colored areas indicate blood flow, signaling the increased blood velocity associated with a cancerous growth.

TREATMENT OF AXILLARY DISEASE

If disease is found in the axillary lymph nodes, there are two main options for treatment: radical radiotherapy and full Level III axillary clearance. Both give good results, but studies have shown that complete axillary clearance gives lower recurrence rates. It provides more information about ultimate outlook and the need for adjuvant therapy, and it avoids the skin irritation and scarring of radiotherapy. The differences, however, are not dramatic, and a 95 percent control rate up to 10 years is possible using radiotherapy.

Although surgeons may feel zealous about clearing every scrap of cancerous tissue from a woman's body, those women who have radiotherapy *and* axillary surgery suffer as a result. Complications include lymphedema (see p.194), damage to the nerves in the axilla, and a reduction in the range of movement in the shoulder. The aim of treating the axilla must therefore be to control disease with the minimum number of postoperative complications.

SURGERY

Level I, II, or III may be indicated, depending on your risk for lymphatic spread. If all Level I nodes are negative, then it is likely that those in Levels II and III will be too. In tumors with low risk of metastatic spread, taking a sample of the Level I nodes may be adequate to ascertain that the axilla is clear, whereas with more high-risk tumors, it may be necessary to sample the nodes at Levels II or III as well.

If you are having a lumpectomy, partial mastectomy, or total mastectomy for invasive breast cancer, you should have an axillary clearance, thus avoiding the need for postoperative radiotherapy of the axilla. This is particularly important when you've opted for immediate breast reconstruction (see p.189), as radiotherapy will significantly affect the cosmetic result.

It may seem like a contradiction that we remove the lymph nodes when their purpose is to fight disease, but in medical terms it makes sense. If they have been infiltrated by cancer, they are no longer effective in any case.

THE PLACE OF RADIOTHERAPY

In the US, the axilla is always treated. The medical world is somewhat divided as to whether the treatment should involve surgery, radiotherapy, or both. If radiotherapy is carried out without surgery having determined that the cancer has spread to the axilla, there is the possibility that women without axillary disease will be exposed to unnecessary radiation. However, although we know that fewer than half the women diagnosed with breast cancer have axillary spread, there is no way to be sure about who is at risk, and therefore everyone gets some treatment.

RECURRENCE IN THE AXILLA

Do discuss the way your doctors intend to treat your axilla, bearing in mind how mobile you want to be and whether or not you would like to have breast reconstruction. With involved axillary nodes, surgical clearance will give you a lower chance of recurrence than radiotherapy alone.

The best treatment
For women with no cancer in the lymph nodes there is only a small difference in rates of recurrence between surgical clearance of the axilla and radiotherapy. For women with involved nodes, however, axillary clearance gives a significantly lower rate of recurrence, making it the treatment of choice.

AXILLARY STATUS	TREATMENT GIVEN	RISK OF RECURRENCE
Node-positive	*Mastectomy and axillary clearance*	*1 percent*
	Mastectomy and radiotherapy to axilla (nodes not cleared)	*12 percent*
Node-negative	*Mastectomy and axillary clearance*	*1½ percent*
	Mastectomy and radiotherapy to axilla (nodes not cleared)	*3 percent*

ADJUVANT THERAPY

Most women with breast cancer will have some form of surgery to remove the tumor, either by taking out the lump alone or by removing the whole breast. By the time the breast cancer is diagnosed, however, some of the cells may have spread beyond the lump itself, so there is a risk that some cancer cells may be left behind after surgery.

In about 40 percent of cases where a cancer appears to involve only a single site within one breast there may be other areas of change in the same breast that are either premalignant or already cancerous. We know that, even when the spread of the tumor is not detectable, in many cases spread to distant parts of the body has already occurred because secondaries appear later on. It may be that small deposits of cancer cells (micrometastases) have spread through the body via the bloodstream and the lymphatic system in up to 70 percent of cases by the time a cancer can be felt.

If these cells are allowed to grow, cancer could come back at the same site (local recurrence) or could spread to form secondary tumors elsewhere in the body (metastases). For this reason, additional forms of treatment (adjuvant therapy) are often given as an insurance policy to destroy remaining cancer cells, wherever they are. There are three main forms of adjuvant treatment:

• radiotherapy given to the breast area to reduce the risk of local recurrence

• hormonal treatment

• chemotherapy (cytotoxic drugs)

Chemotherapy and hormone treatment are aimed at reducing the risk of secondary growth (metastases) elsewhere in the body. These are both called *systemic* treatments. Some form of systemic treatment is probably advisable for most patients, even after surgery and radiotherapy combined, because the odds of dying in any year can be lowered by 25 percent. After 10 years, 3 in 10 deaths could be avoided in the US, and in the UK 2,000 lives every year could be saved by using systemic adjuvant therapy.

Ideally, an anticancer therapy should be able to kill off only cells affected by the disease without harming healthy cells. Unfortunately, no anticancer treatment is that discriminating, so some healthy cells are bound to be affected, sometimes leading to side effects (see p.187). Discuss side effects with your doctor before deciding to proceed with any treatment.

RADIOTHERAPY

Adjuvant radiotherapy is given to catch any cancer cells that may have been left behind after surgery. We now know that simple mastectomy plus local radiotherapy is just as effective a treatment as radical mastectomy, both in terms of controlling local spread and survival rates. A very large UK study involving nearly 3,000 women showed that there was no difference in survival rates between the two treatments, but showed a marked improvement in controlling local recurrence in women who received radiotherapy. The risk of local recurrence in women who were not treated with radiotherapy was approximately three times greater than the risk in those who were.

At one time radiotherapy was standard treatment after all mastectomies, but now doctors are more selective. If you fulfill any of the following criteria you may be a candidate for postoperative radiotherapy:

- a large tumor – more than 2 inches (5 centimeters) in diameter
- more than 4 positive nodes
- certain localized metastatic breast cancers

Even so, deciding who gets radiotherapy is not a cut-and-dried procedure, because only about a third of women are at risk of recurrence, so many women would receive unnecessary doses of radiotherapy if all patients were treated.

There's no doubt that radiotherapy should be given to all high-risk women who have aggressive tumors. For women at lower risk – those with a small, node-negative tumor, for example – it may be safe to monitor closely and use radiotherapy only if the cancer returns. Though your hopes may be dashed by local recurrence, try not to get too depressed, as it does not seem to affect long-term survival rates anyway, provided you get radiotherapy at the time.

HOW RADIOTHERAPY IS GIVEN

The aim of adjuvant radiation treatment is to ensure that all the cancer cells in the area of the affected breast are destroyed, or in the case of localized metastatic cancers, to relieve pain in the affected area. For cancer in the breast, doses of high-energy X-rays are accurately beamed at the breast area of the chest wall and occasionally the axilla and the area above the collarbone. An average course of radiotherapy involves five out-patient treatments a week over about six weeks. Each dose of radiation is meticulously calculated and is then precisely delivered to the area of your skin that will have been marked with a tiny tattoo or blue dye. Each session can take several minutes, during which time you will have to lie very still. Otherwise, the experience is not different from that of having an ordinary X-ray. You will be asked not to wash the area during the treatment to avoid irritating the skin. Radiation treatment will not make you radioactive, and there is no danger to children or adults from coming into contact with you.

A BOOSTER DOSE OF RADIATION

We know that tumors tend to recur within their margins, which is why surgeons will take about 1 centimeter of healthy breast tissue all around the tumor. When performing a lumpectomy, your

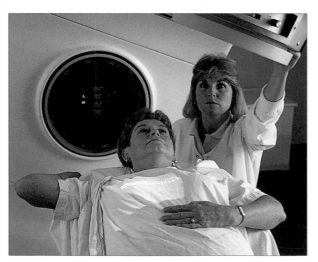

Radiotherapy session
This woman is about to have radiation treatment. Her right arm is raised, since the treatment is for her right breast. The radiotherapist sets up the machine, then leaves the room during the actual treatment.

surgeon faces the dilemma of taking as little normal tissue as possible to retain the shape of your breast, at the same time removing enough tissue to ensure maximum safety. Some surgeons feel they can strike the optimum compromise if a booster dose of radiation is given to smash any remaining cancer cells.

The boost can be given in several ways, but common to all methods is the delivery of a large dose of extra radiation in a short time. In Europe and the US, many centers use electron therapy, which is very precise and leaves the lungs unharmed. Other centers have tried implanting tubes at the site of surgery, which can be loaded with radioactive material after the operation. At first iridium was used, but cesium has superseded it. This has proved to be a very labor-intensive procedure involving specially designated treatment areas and therefore is not practiced widely. The booster dose is given in addition to the standard course of radiotherapy.

SIDE EFFECTS OF RADIATION

Serious side effects are rare with modern techniques. Radiotherapy to the breast area does not cause infertility, nor will your hair fall out. You could find the treatments very tiring, so it's a good idea to put aside rest time on your return from the hospital and to be relaxed about routine chores.

Any side effects will usually subside within a few weeks of your stopping radiotherapy, and by no means everyone experiences them. Don't expose the treated skin to the sun for about 18 months.

• Occasionally sickness follows treatment, and meals may have to be planned carefully around sessions.

• Skin exposed to radiotherapy may become darker, slightly itchy, and sore as though sunburned. Women with fair skin, particularly those with red hair, are more likely to have skin problems than are darker-skinned women.

• Small blood vessels in the skin may dilate and burst, forming tiny red marks.

• The top of the lungs may be affected because radiation can cause scarring during treatment, leaving behind a dry cough or breathlessness that may take a few months to clear up. Tangential radiation prevents this.

• In the past, high-dose radiotherapy was given to the axilla, and there was always the danger of painful swelling of the arm (*lymphedema*, see p.194). Nowadays this kind of radiotherapy is rarely used.

• Radiotherapy has the potential to interfere with the body's immune system, but with modern dosing this side effect is very rare.

SYSTEMIC ADJUVANT TREATMENT

The word *systemic* means affecting the whole. Systemic adjuvant therapy aims to kill off cancer cells throughout your body, thereby preventing any cells that have migrated from the original tumor from causing metastases in the lungs, liver, and bones. The type of systemic treatment that you're eligible for is

STATUS	TREATMENT
Premenopausal, node-negative	*None or tamoxifen (high-risk women may have chemotherapy or ovarian treatment recommended)*
Premenopausal, node-positive	*Adjuvant chemotherapy*
Postmenopausal, node-negative	*Tamoxifen for most patients in this group*
Postmenopausal, node-positive	*Tamoxifen; chemotherapy will be considered if the tumor is aggressive*

Summary of systemic adjuvant therapy
Two main factors determine what kind of systemic therapy will be used to treat breast cancer: whether you are pre- or postmenopausal, and whether the cancer has spread to the axillary nodes.

largely determined by your age (see chart, left). If you are under 50, chemotherapy has been shown to have the most dramatic effect in reducing your odds of dying from the cancer. If you are post-menopausal, hormone treatment in the form of tamoxifen has the same life-saving effect when used for at least two years, especially in tumors that are hormone-sensitive.

HORMONE TREATMENT

Breast cancers may sometimes be influenced by the levels and fluctuations of a woman's hormones, and so lowering estrogen levels in a woman's body may help to combat some forms of breast cancer. A few breast cancers are very sensitive to estrogen levels, and so the various forms of hormone treatment are aimed at reducing or abolishing a woman's estrogen production. These treatments include:

• the use of antiestrogen drugs such as tamoxifen

• surgical removal of the ovaries or their destruction by X-rays

• treatment with drugs to stop estrogen production

Tamoxifen The first option is tamoxifen, a drug that blocks the stimulatory effect of estrogen on breast-cancer cells. It may also have other actions – stimulating the body's own natural anticancer defenses, for example. Over the last ten years tamoxifen has produced a modest but extremely exciting breakthrough in breast-cancer treatment. One 20-milligram tablet taken daily for between two and five years offers a 20–30 percent reduction in the risk of dying from breast cancer. This appears to continue for at least ten years.

Tamoxifen, although it slightly increases the risk of uterine cancer and should not be used after thrombosis, has few side effects apart from causing menopausal symptoms in some premenopausal women. Like natural estrogen, it reduces the risk of heart disease and prevents postmenopausal bone loss (osteoporosis).

The benefits of tamoxifen apply to all women irrespective of their age or the stage of their cancer, but women over the age of 50 and who have estrogen-receptor-positive tumors seem to gain most. The majority of postmenopausal women are therefore given tamoxifen for at least two years after breast-cancer surgery irrespective of grade, stage, or lymph-node involvement.

The role of tamoxifen in premenopausal women is less certain, and the best adjuvant treatment for younger women is still debated. Tamoxifen could play an increasingly important role in the prevention of breast cancer (see p.153).

Destruction of the ovaries (ablation) Abolishing the secretion of estrogen by the ovaries with either surgery or radiotherapy has been shown to give about a 10 percent increase in overall survival rate for premenopausal women with breast cancer. It also reduces the number of women who get a recurrence by about 25 percent. Specialists prefer to use ablation in only those younger women at very high risk; immediate menopause and infertility result.

Goserelin An alternative approach is to inject goserelin, which inhibits brain hormones that control the ovaries' output of estrogen. This reduction in estrogen levels may cause menopausal symptoms in premenopausal women. These effects are reversible when treatment is stopped. The treatment will continue, depending on its efficacy and side effects.

CHEMOTHERAPY

Whereas tamoxifen is primarily a treatment for postmenopausal women, chemotherapy is used mainly in younger women. Cytotoxic drugs find and kill cancer cells anywhere in the body and are often given after breast-cancer surgery, particularly to premenopausal women whose axillary lymph nodes are involved or whose tumors are particularly aggressive. Chemotherapy will delay relapse by 30 percent and lower the risk of dying by up to 25 percent.

If you do not want surgery or your tumor is unsuitable for surgery, chemotherapy may be the first or only treatment. There are many different kinds of anticancer drugs that are used in different combinations, and their success rates and side effects may differ from woman to woman. Prolonged multiple drug treatment – cyclical combination chemotherapy in the form of CMF (cyclophosphamide, methotrexate, and 5-fluorouracil) or CAF (cyclophosphamide, adriamycin, and 5-fluorouracil) – is most used. CAF is used with younger women and those with greater risk of recurrence, CMF with older women or those unable to tolerate CAF.

In France chemotherapy is being used preoperatively, since recent research suggests that chemotherapy before surgery may improve survival rates. Clinical trials comparing pre- and postoperative chemotherapy have started, and if this approach proves favorable, chemotherapy before surgery may become more popular. The use of hormone treatment plus anticancer drugs in combination may be more effective than either treatment alone, and this regimen is also being tested in clinical trials.

Treatment Adjuvant chemotherapy is usually given by injection or through a drip inserted into a vein in your arm. Treatment tends to be given in cycles at monthly intervals for six months. Although outpatient treatment is possible, a hospital stay overnight after each treatment is not a bad idea, so that any side effects can be dealt with quickly.

Side effects of chemotherapy The most worrisome effect of chemotherapy is possible damage to the bone marrow, which replenishes blood cells; white cells are the most vulnerable. To check that levels of white blood cells remain normal and the body's defenses against infection are intact, a blood sample will be taken before each treatment. If the white-cell count is too low, your next course of treatment will be put off or the dose reduced until the white-cell count returns to a safe level. To ameliorate these side effects, antibiotics or a blood transfusion during a course of chemotherapy are sometimes required.

Other side effects include tiredness, nausea, some hair loss, mouth ulcers, loss of appetite, and diarrhea. Any or all of these can make you feel miserable and ill. Simple remedies such as mouthwashes can help to combat mouth soreness, and powerful anti-emetic drugs have been specially developed to stop the nausea associated with the treatment. If your appetite is affected by treatment, whether it is suppressed or your weight begins to increase, your doctor or special-care nurse will be able to give you dietary advice. Some foods have been found to react with anticancer drugs, but this is rare.

Certain drugs will have different effects on hair loss. With CMF, you may experience little or no loss. CAF, on the other hand, is more likely to result in hair loss. For some women this is the most distressing side effect, especially coming on top of the trauma of disfiguring breast surgery. Your hair will grow back after treatment or even before the treatment is finished, but it may be a little more curly and may change color slightly.

Menstruation can often be disrupted by anticancer drugs and may stop altogether. About 40 percent of women who are treated with chemotherapy will become infertile, and you should discuss the possibility with your doctor before treatment begins. The younger you are, the more likely your periods are to restart when chemotherapy ends.

STEM CELL TREATMENT

About 15 years ago it appeared that women with advanced breast cancer who received very high doses of cytotoxic agents were likely to live longer. Doses, however, are constrained by the poisonous effect on bone marrow. To combat this, researchers developed a procedure called autologous stem cell transfusion, which uses the woman's own bone marrow to rescue her from otherwise toxic high doses of chemotherapy. At this time the procedure remains controversial, traumatic, and very expensive, and unfortunately it is not as successful as was first hoped.

Stem cells, the cells that produce all other blood cells, are removed from the patient's blood or bone marrow and frozen. Then a course of high-dose chemotherapy is given over a period of 4–5 days in doses that would usually be sufficient to kill the stem cells, leading ultimately to the patient's death. Having taken the precaution of saving some of the stem cells from injury, however, doctors can reinfuse them after chemotherapy is complete. Because these cells have not been affected by chemotherapy, they can once again begin to form healthy blood cells.

Stem cell treatment can be had in some centers in the US, but rarely in Europe. Clinical trials are underway on both sides of the Atlantic to compare it with conventional chemotherapy. Most centers await publication of the results before offering the procedure. Some medical insurance or HMO plans do not cover experimental treatments.

BREAST RECONSTRUCTION

If you have lost part or all of your breast, you can have reconstructive surgery. This involves the creation of a natural-looking artificial breast through plastic surgery. Although a reconstructed breast may look very real, there will be little or no feeling in the transferred skin. The psychological benefits and increased confidence you will experience in the way you look tend to outweigh the disadvantage of reduced sensation of the nipple and areola.

Every woman has the right to consult a specialist about reconstruction. If your doctor is reluctant to consider the option, seek a second opinion. Even the most well-adjusted woman flinches at the thought of a mastectomy. It's reasonable to see the changes you have to make to the way you dress and to your lifestyle as a threat to your femininity and body image. Above all, the mastectomy scar may serve as a reminder of the cancer you once had. Reconstruction can go a long way to making you feel whole again. You will no longer need prostheses (false breasts) or special bras. Nor will you feel so restricted in the kind of clothes that you wear. Reconstruction can contribute a great deal to your self-esteem and your optimism about the future. About half of all mastectomy patients choose to have breast reconstruction, finding that it helps them to put their cancer behind them.

Reconstruction in no way restricts the various treatments that are available to you. It does not interfere with radiotherapy, chemotherapy, or hormone therapy. Postoperative follow-up is made no more difficult, and recurrence can still be detected easily.

TIMING

Some consideration should be given to the timing of reconstruction. It may be possible for you to have it immediately after your mastectomy and under the same anesthetic, or at any time afterward. This means that a woman who had a mastectomy many years ago when breast reconstruction was not available can opt to have it now.

With immediate reconstruction you will wake from your operation with your breast still present even though it will have altered. The psychological stress associated with breast removal is greatly reduced, and in addition, you don't have to cope with the prospect of more surgery later.

These advantages have made immediate reconstruction standard in about 90 percent of surgically treated breast cancers in the US. This procedure involves two specialists – the cancer surgeon and the plastic surgeon – working at the same time. There are different ways to perform the reconstruction – with implants, expanders, and flaps of skin, fat, and muscle from your own body. Discuss your options with your plastic surgeon before making your choice. Ask about the risks and benefits of each procedure for you in particular

You may not be able to take advantage of immediate reconstruction in the clinic that you attend, but, if this is what you want, it may be possible to be transferred to a center that does offer it.

WHO IS SUITABLE FOR RECONSTRUCTION?

Don't worry if you are slightly unfit – reconstructive surgery can be performed on any woman except the very frail. Even if you have widespread disease you may still have a life expectancy of several years, and the quality of your life during this time can be greatly improved by reconstruction.

Although half of all breast-cancer patients will not need a mastectomy, even women who have conservative surgery may lose quite a lot of breast tissue. They too can take advantage of reconstructive surgery.

METHODS OF RECONSTRUCTION

Reconstructive surgery remolds your breast mound, areola, and nipple. The mound can be reconstructed using your own tissue (fat and muscle) or an artificial implant. The implant can be silicone or a saline-filled sac (see p.113).

ARTIFICIAL IMPLANTS

A fixed-volume implant is placed behind the pectoralis muscle in exactly the same way as for breast augmentation (see p.111–12). Although this is the simplest operation, it's not suitable for all women, as there may not be enough skin in the breast area to accommodate the implant.

An alternative is an expander implant, which may be recommended if too little skin remains after your mastectomy to cover a fixed-volume implant. An expander implant – an empty sac with a hollow tube and small valve attached – is placed behind the pectoralis muscle. Over a period of several months, your doctor will gradually fill the implant with saline solution, allowing the skin to stretch so that a fixed-volume implant may eventually be inserted.

YOUR OWN TISSUE

There are several methods of reconstruction using your own tissue, all of them involving "flaps." Skin, muscle, and fat are taken from either your back (latissimus dorsi flap) or your abdomen (rectus abdominis) – also known as the TRAM (transverse rectus abdominis myocutaneous) flap. Tissues with their arteries and veins intact are swiveled up to your breast area so that they can "take" in a similar way to a skin graft. The flap is tunneled underneath your skin to the breast area and is fashioned into a breast mound resembling your other breast as closely as possible. Many women find these implants preferable to the artificial varieties. These reconstructions require quite complex surgery, and occasionally there are side effects, such as a weakening of the abdominal muscles if a large amount of tissue has to be moved.

The final type of reconstruction is one that uses a free flap, for instance one that takes tissue from your abdomen (rectus abdominis flap) or your buttocks (free gluteus flap). In this case blood vessels supplying the tissue that is moved are cut and rejoined to blood vessels in the chest wall where the implant is placed. This is the most complex kind of reconstruction, and for some patients it may be the most satisfactory. There is a small risk that the blood vessels will fail to join, in which case the implant may not take.

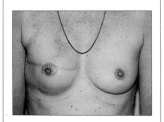

Reconstructed breast
In this example of a reconstruction, both the right breast and nipple have been reconstructed after a total mastectomy.

RECONSTRUCTION PROCEDURES

The simplest kind of reconstruction is carried out
with an implant. The more complex "flap"
operations, however, produce a better result.

EXPANDER IMPLANT

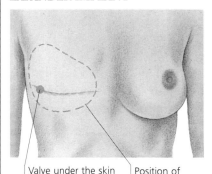

Valve under the skin
allows saline to be
injected later | Position of
expander
under skin

*A hollow sac with a valve is put in
place. Over a period of months,
saline fluid is injected into the valve,
so the skin can stretch gradually. The
expander can then be replaced with
a fixed-volume implant.*

LATISSIMUS DORSI FLAP

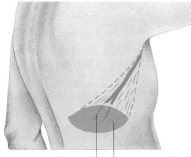

Blood vessels
not cut | Section of skin,
muscle, and fat
to be moved

*1 A flap of skin, muscle, and fat is
taken from the latissimus dorsi
muscle on the back. The section of
tissue to be moved keeps its feeding
artery intact even after it has been
moved to the new site.*

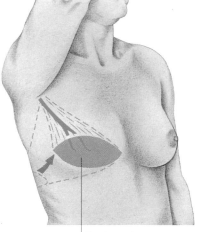

Flap brought
under skin to
front of chest

*2 The flap is tunneled under the
skin to the site of the mastectomy
scar, and the fat and muscle are
fashioned into a breast mound. The
new breast is sewn into place, and
the incision in the back is closed.*

RECTUS ABDOMINIS FLAP

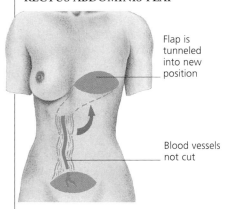

Flap is
tunneled
into new
position

Blood vessels
not cut

*The flap is taken from the rectus
abdominis muscle with its blood
supply intact. It is tunneled under
the skin to its new position. The
incision in the abdomen is closed
and the new breast mound stitched
into place.*

FREE GLUTEUS FLAP

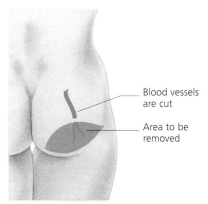

Blood vessels
are cut

Area to be
removed

*1 A flap of skin, muscle, and fat is
taken from the gluteus maximus
muscle in the buttocks. The feeding
artery to the flap is severed so the
flap can simply be placed in position
without having to be tunneled under
the skin as for other methods.*

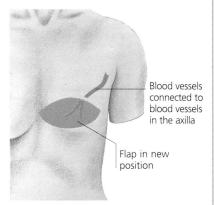

Blood vessels
connected to
blood vessels
in the axilla

Flap in new
position

*2 The flap is transferred to
the mastectomy area, and
microsurgery is used to connect the
blood vessels to the vessels behind
the muscles in the chest. The flap
is then stitched into place, and the
incision in the buttocks is closed.*

THE IMPACT OF TREATMENT

Over the past 40 years, surgeons have performed far less radical breast surgery, yet the diagnosis of breast cancer and its treatment – especially if it involves the loss of a breast – still brings havoc in its wake. Psychiatric disturbance is approximately three times more likely following mastectomy than in the general population of women. Despite the advent of breast-conserving techniques, rates of anxiety and depression are still high. Women are just as anxious about having cancer as they are about the potential loss of breast.

Nor are the psychological problems necessarily less if you have a lumpectomy rather than a mastectomy. For doctors to believe that your fears are minor compared with those of a woman facing a mastectomy could cause problems that may continue throughout your treatment, even into the follow-up period. Your feeling that you shouldn't bother your doctors with your fears may also be a reflection of conditioning that expects women to be unreasonably stoical in the face of both physical and emotional pain.

A woman with breast cancer who's had a lumpectomy shouldn't be required to handle the disease with cheerfulness and fortitude. Nor should just having a "little lump" removed create the feeling that, as treatment was comparatively trivial, you should quickly return to a normal psychological state; if you can't, you could end up feeling worthless and depressed.

A preoperative psychological test can reveal 90 percent of women who will become anxious and depressed in the year following surgery, enabling proper follow-up and help to be offered. If you feel vulnerable, ask for a test using the HAD (Hospital Anxiety and Depression) scale.

RADIOTHERAPY

Radiotherapy can involve daily treatment for up to six weeks. The greater the amount of radiation, the greater the chance of side effects, which can be draining. Although you may worry that radiation will prevent you from having children, the radiated area is far from the ovaries and they are not affected by the treatment. When doctors try to help with comments like "It's an insurance policy just to be sure we have gotten all the cancer," they sometimes create doubt rather than reassuring you. Just the thought of having radiotherapy can sometimes be sufficient to produce side effects. The more you understand about your treatment, the less anxious you will be.

CHEMOTHERAPY

Chemotherapy has the worst reputation of all breast-cancer treatments, as it's nearly always followed by some side effects, from nausea and hair loss to an increased risk of infection.

For a woman who is feeling emotionally and physically bruised, the prospect of going through several courses of chemotherapy can cause a mixture of fear and suspicion. As with radiotherapy, the need for chemotherapy sometimes provokes fears that the cancer has not been totally removed.

Understandably you will become more anxious and depressed if you have troublesome side effects. Don't be afraid to disclose the extent of your suffering to doctors for fear that life-saving treatment will be stopped. It's a mistake to believe that a treatment must hurt to be effective. You should never suffer in silence; tell your caregivers about your distress and discomfort, and they will do all they can to give you the help and support you need.

BODY IMAGE

Far too often decisions about treatment are based on assumptions that older women or the sexually inactive won't mind losing a breast. In one study of 62 women more than half of those who chose lumpectomy were over the age of 50 and more than a quarter were over 60, demonstrating that age is not an acceptable criterion for deciding treatment.

You may become extremely self-conscious following mastectomy. Some women feel sure that people can tell they have only one breast, and become so distressed they withdraw from the company of other people. Up to a third of postmastectomy patients are unhappy with their prosthesis.

Although mastectomy clearly has the greatest impact on body image, not every woman who has breast conservation is pleased with the cosmetic outcome. Some women feel that being told they would have only the lump removed was misleading, as they expected to be left with symmetrical breasts. Unfortunately, wide local excision does not always fulfill these ideals.

SEXUAL RELATIONSHIPS

Powerful sexual stereotyping in our society means that breasts have become symbolically linked to motherhood, femininity, and sexuality. Don't feel inadequate if breast loss causes you severe sexual disturbance with lowered self-esteem, loss of perceived attractiveness, embarrassment or inhibition, and loss of sex drive. About 1 in 5 women has a loss of sexual interest a few months after mastectomy, and at two years the figure rises to 1 in 3.

Interest in sex declines in over a quarter of sexually active women irrespective of the kind of surgical treatment they have. If you have had adjuvant therapy, you are particularly vulnerable and likely to express more concern about physical affection, sexual relationships, and lost feelings of femininity or sexual attractiveness. You may lose a lot of sensation in the affected breast following radiotherapy, and your partner may seem reluctant to touch the breast.

If your breasts were an important source of sexual stimulation prior to surgery, then you will need help and counseling to find another means of enhancing your enjoyment of lovemaking. Your partner may worry about being exposed to radiation by touching your breast while you are undergoing radiotherapy. This is not a danger.

The psychological impact of the diagnosis of cancer and treatment may make you so overwhelmingly preoccupied with thoughts of survival that sexual desire is at the bottom of your list of priorities. For some couples, however, the trauma of breast cancer can bring them closer together.

My husband was just great, really supportive. I know that he was far more worried that I had a life-threatening disease than about the loss of my breast. But our sex life has changed, of course it has. I can't rid myself of the idea that really he hates my scar but is just trying to pretend that he doesn't mind.

CHERYL, 36, MUSICIAN

LIFE AFTER TREATMENT

When treatment for breast cancer is complete, the story does not simply end. Rigorous follow-up will be necessary to pick up any problems and to check for recurrence of the cancer. Having a mastectomy means that there are adjustments to make: you have to get used to a prosthesis and exercises to make your arm muscles strong. Then you have to learn to live with your new body. Even when treatment is complete, you could have psychological difficulties. After months of intensive medical attention you may feel alone and fearful, especially knowing there is no guarantee of a cure. This is a time when a care network such as a local breast-cancer group can be invaluable.

LYMPHEDEMA

Disfigurement caused by surgery is not the only possible trauma you may face. Lymphedema, painful swelling of the arm caused by radical radiotherapy or surgery on the axilla, can occasionally arise after treatment.

Healthy lymph nodes act as filters for the lymph fluid. Surgery can cause scarring of the nodes, resulting in a blockage of the drainage system. The fluid stagnates in the arm, causing swelling and stiffness, and may be accompanied by a painful shoulder and possibly by nerve pain. With modern surgical techniques lymphedema is rare now, and only 5 percent of mastectomy patients suffer from it to any degree. Severe lymphedema hardly ever occurs.

Prevention and treatment After the removal of your lymph nodes you become more susceptible to infection, so you should protect your arm from knocks and scrapes and wear gloves for rough household chores, gardening, or any other work in which your skin could be chafed.

It's important to perform your postmastectomy exercises (see p.196), as this can help to reduce the swelling by encouraging lymph drainage. Whenever you can, keep your arm raised, even in bed or sitting on a sofa. Put your arm on a pile of cushions to keep it at about the same level as your neck. This will reduce swelling in your arm and help to maintain the good work achieved by your daily exercises. If you have problems overnight with tingling in the fingers, try wearing an elastic bandage to prevent your arm from swelling.

PROSTHESES

A prosthesis is a false breast without a nipple but with an axillary tail so that in all respects it resembles the texture, fullness, and shape of a real breast. You will be able to wear a lightweight, temporary one as soon as your scar is healed and then be fitted with a permanent one to fit comfortably into your bra.

Every woman has the right to a good prosthesis. With the help of your surgeon or breast-care nurse, you should easily be able to obtain one and even try various types to find the one that feels right. In the best hospitals you will find a specially trained counselor who will advise you about the suitability of different kinds of prostheses and how to wear them.

If at first you can't find a prosthesis that's right for you, don't be disheartened. No prosthesis can fully replace your breast, but there is a good prosthesis for every woman who has had a mastectomy. There are many that will allow you to wear a swimsuit and low necklines without anyone being the wiser, and you will soon feel quite confident with your new shape. (There is a range of prostheses for women whose breasts are asymmetrical following conservative surgery, and these are quite discreet.)

CHOOSING BRAS

When your permanent prosthesis has been fitted, there's no reason why you shouldn't wear a wide variety of bras. The exceptions include bras that are wide and low-cut, such as a half-cup bra. It's best to choose a cotton bra so sweat can evaporate and your skin doesn't become sticky under the prosthesis.

There are many attractive bras available with specially fitted pockets to hold your prosthesis in place, ensuring that it does not slip. Extra support in the rib-band and wide, supportive shoulder straps are important for comfort and can help your posture, which can be affected by a mastectomy.

BREAST PROSTHESES

A permanent prosthesis is made from silicone. It "gives" to the touch and feels heavy, just like a normal breast. Lightweight prostheses can be useful as a temporary measure, for night wear and sports, or for very hot days when a permanent prosthesis can feel sticky and uncomfortable.

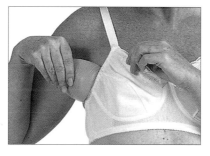

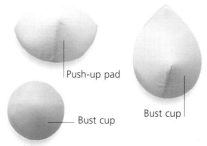

Push-up pad

Bust cup

Bust cup

SILICONE PROSTHESIS
Soft to the touch, a silicone prosthesis has the weight and droop of a natural breast.

Silicone nipples adhere to prosthesis when moistened

FITTING A PROSTHESIS
The prosthesis simply slips into the pocket inside your bra. Make sure that it fills the cup and that your underarm area is filled to the same extent on both sides.

BRA FILLERS
A variety of push-up pads and bust cups are available to fill out your bra after partial mastectomy.

LIGHTWEIGHT PROSTHESIS
This foam prosthesis has a hollow back that allows air to circulate and is light and comfortable to wear.

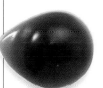

Prostheses can be tinted to skin color

Triangular form for less radical surgery

Underarm extension for extensive surgery

Teardrop shape fills bra up to strap

Lightweight form for night wear

POSTMASTECTOMY EXERCISES

You may find that your shoulder movement is restricted immediately following your operation. Normal movement and flexibility should gradually return, however, with the help of a few simple exercises.

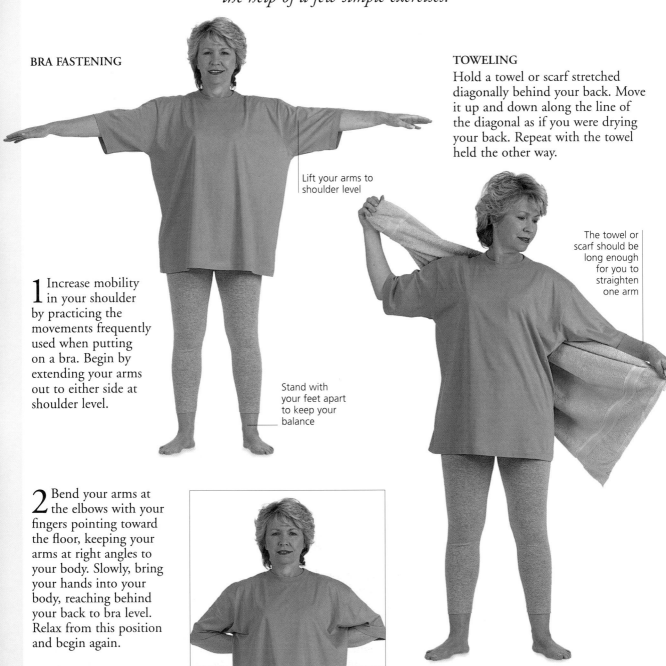

BRA FASTENING

1 Increase mobility in your shoulder by practicing the movements frequently used when putting on a bra. Begin by extending your arms out to either side at shoulder level.

Lift your arms to shoulder level

Stand with your feet apart to keep your balance

2 Bend your arms at the elbows with your fingers pointing toward the floor, keeping your arms at right angles to your body. Slowly, bring your hands into your body, reaching behind your back to bra level. Relax from this position and begin again.

TOWELING

Hold a towel or scarf stretched diagonally behind your back. Move it up and down along the line of the diagonal as if you were drying your back. Repeat with the towel held the other way.

The towel or scarf should be long enough for you to straighten one arm

HAIR BRUSHING

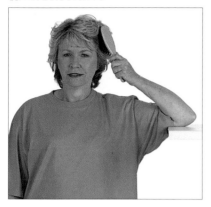

Rest your arm on a firm surface. Keeping your head and shoulders upright, brush your hair upward and sideways.

HAND SQUEEZES

Hold a rubber ball or similar object in the palm of your hand. The ball should be firm enough for you to have to exert pressure to squeeze it, but should give enough for you to notice any improvement in muscle strength. Forming a fist around the ball, gently squeeze, then release. Repeat the exercise, but stop if you begin to ache.

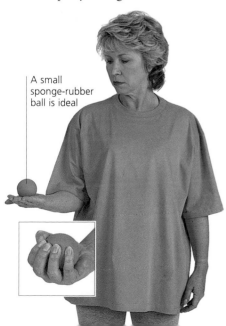

A small sponge-rubber ball is ideal

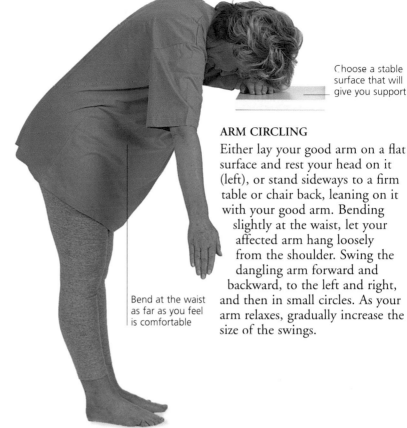

Choose a stable surface that will give you support

Bend at the waist as far as you feel is comfortable

ARM CIRCLING

Either lay your good arm on a flat surface and rest your head on it (left), or stand sideways to a firm table or chair back, leaning on it with your good arm. Bending slightly at the waist, let your affected arm hang loosely from the shoulder. Swing the dangling arm forward and backward, to the left and right, and then in small circles. As your arm relaxes, gradually increase the size of the swings.

WALL REACHING

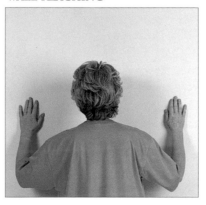

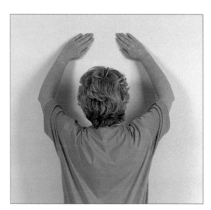

1 This will increase the mobility in your shoulder. Stand facing a wall with your feet apart for balance. Place the palms of your hands flat against the wall at shoulder height. Be careful not to lean your weight on your arms.

2 Slowly begin to work your hands up the wall, but stop if you feel any discomfort. Slide them back to shoulder level and begin again. Aim to reach higher than previously, to increase your flexibility, but do not overstretch.

RECURRENCE AND RISK

Your age, menopausal status, the stage of the disease, and the status of your axillary nodes will all have a profound affect on your initial chances of survival. In very general terms, women developing breast cancer under the age of 35 do not fare so well as those whose breast cancer starts around the time of menopause. Women between the ages of 35 and 50 who have not yet started menopause do best. This still means that many, many women have a good chance of surviving breast cancer, especially if it is detected early.

After successful treatment for breast cancer you will be concerned about how carefully you'll be followed up and how long it will be before you can be considered cured. The longer you live without a recurrence, the longer you will remain cancer-free and the higher the chances of a cure. Because of this, most doctors believe that you should be carefully monitored for at least five years after treatment to detect possible recurrences or secondary spread.

You must be followed up for longer than five years before you can be said to be cured. Survival beyond 10 years without any evidence of recurrence or spread would lead a doctor to be optimistic that you were cured, although women who have had breast cancer in the past may still have a very small increased chance of dying from it, even 40 years after treatment, compared with healthy women of the same age.

TREATMENT FOR RECURRENCE

Cancer can recur in the area of the treated breast regardless of your initial treatment. This happens in 2 or 3 cases out of 10, but is not a reason to be terrified or despondent. Radiotherapy can cure any local recurrence, which is why follow-up schedules for patients must be strictly adhered to. A recurrence can then be detected so early that a relatively small dose of radiotherapy is all that is needed to eradicate it. We have to remember that there is a difference between the frequency of local recurrence after mastectomy and lumpectomy, the former being slightly lower. Lumpectomy has a recurrence rate of 10–30 percent, whereas with mastectomy it's 5–15 percent. In addition, radiotherapy following a lumpectomy is often given at the total body dose, so it is no longer an option for treating a recurrence.

TYPES OF RECURRENCE

There are three ways in which cancer can recur in the breast area. The most common recurrence is in the conserved breast in the region of the original cancer. This is not necessarily too serious – it's seen as cancer that is left over from the original treatment rather than a secondary metastasis. Because the cancer has not spread around the body, this type of recurrence is usually treated with a mastectomy.

Although rare, affecting only 2 percent of women, another kind of local recurrence concerns the lymph nodes. In general this is not considered to be a sign of metastasis and is therefore treated with further surgery or radiation.

A recurrence in the scar or chest wall following a mastectomy is more serious. Because all your breast tissue has been removed, it is impossible for the cancer to be residual, and therefore it must have traveled from the lymphatic system or the bloodstream. Such recurrence, or recurrence in your other breast or elsewhere in your body, is considered a metastasis and will certainly require rigorous attention to curb the spreading cancer.

PREVIOUS BREAST CANCER AND RISK

A woman who has already had cancer of one breast is at a higher than average risk of developing cancer of the other breast, and this is why women who have had breast cancer must be meticulous about carrying out BSE on their remaining breast. Tamoxifen (see p.186) seems to reduce the risk of a second cancer developing regardless of whether adjuvant treatment has been given, and in women with several risk factors, prophylactic (preventive) tamoxifen might be considered. You should discuss this with your doctor.

As well as carrying out BSE for yourself, you should also have regular mammograms performed on your remaining breast, because about 7 out of 100 women may develop a second primary tumor at some time in the future. A reasonable schedule for follow-up mammography would be twice a year for two years and every 12 months thereafter.

THE REMAINING BREAST

There has been an interesting study performed on women under 65 with Stage I or Stage II breast cancers – in other words, early cancer. When biopsy was performed on the opposite breast, nearly 1 in 6 women were found to have some cancerous changes at the time of finding the first tumor. The vast majority of changes, however, proved to be pre-invasive DCIS (see p.156) – cancers that might never have become symptomatic and certainly would not kill. So these findings are of doubtful significance, and it's still not clear which patients need treatment for them.

Doctors cannot agree whether the opposite breast should be biopsied at the time of initial surgery or during follow-up. Performing these biopsies might detect a good number of in situ lesions that if left alone would cause no problems at all. On the other hand, because only a very small sample of breast tissue is taken during a biopsy, it's possible to miss some invasive cancers that are present. Such obsessive searching for cancers can lead to intense and unnecessary anxiety, and a sensible course to follow seems to be to monitor the remaining breast during follow-up sessions and reserve biopsy for any suspicious physical or mammographic findings. Do not hesitate to discuss with your doctor any uncertainties or worries you may have.

In conclusion, bear in mind that 1 in 3 women who have treatment for early breast cancer can expect to have a normal life span. For women who get local recurrences, radiotherapy can cure without the need for other treatment. Lastly, while breast cancer is predominantly a disease of older women, many women will die from causes other than their breast cancer.

GLOSSARY

The following list includes unfamiliar words that recur throughout this book, or that you may hear used by doctors and medical staff. Many of the terms are explained in more detail in the relevant chapters.

Ablation Destruction by means of X-rays or laser beam.

Adjuvant Additional to, as in adjuvant therapy (see p.183).

Axilla The armpit.

Bilateral Both sides, as in affecting both breasts.

Biopsy Taking a specimen of tissue to make a precise diagnosis (as in cutting-needle biopsy, see p.160).

Calcification Deposits of calcium in a breast lump that show up on mammogram as white dots.

Carcinoma Cancer.

Contracture Hardening of scar tissue around a breast implant.

Cyst A benign, fluid-filled lump.

Cytology Examining cells from a lump or cyst for any evidence of cancer, as in fine-needle aspiration cytology (FNAC, see p.127).

Ectasia Dilatation of the milk ducts behind the nipple.

Fibroadenoma A harmless lump formed during the natural growth cycle of a breast lobule.

Fistula An abnormal opening, such as from a chronic abscess to the skin or into a milk duct (as in nipple fistula).

Galactorrhea The production of milk by a woman who isn't pregnant or lactating.

Granuloma A small lump resulting from chronic inflammation.

Histology The study of tissues under a microscope. The tissue comes from a biopsy specimen.

Hormone A chemical messenger from one part of the body that circulates in the bloodstream and exerts an effect on another part.

Hyperplasia Excessive cell growth.

Impalpable Cannot be felt.

In situ cancer Noninvasive cancer confined to where it arises. It does not spread and it is not fatal.

Involution Dying back, shrinking.

Lesion Any newly formed abnormal structure in the body.

Lobule The glandular part of the breast where milk is produced.

Luteal phase The second half of the menstrual cycle, after ovulation.

Lymph nodes or glands The junctions of the lymphatic system (see p.40) that become enlarged if fighting an infection or cancer.

Lymphedema Swelling, pain, and stiffness of the arm and hand, due to interference with the lymphatic drainage (see p.40) of the axilla following surgery and more often radiotherapy. It is now fairly rare.

Mastitis Inflammation of breast tissue.

Metastasis Spread of a cancer to a distant part of the body where it forms a secondary tumor.

Microcalcifications Minute calcium deposits that have a white speckled appearance on mammography.

Micrometastasis A secondary tumor formed from only one or two cells that have escaped from the primary tumor.

Oncogene A cancer-promoting gene.

Oncology The study of cancer. An oncologist is a specialist in cancer and cancer treatments.

Peau d'orange Literally "orange peel." Dimpling of the skin caused by a breast tumor spreading upward to tether the skin.

Pedicle A stalk.

Prosthesis An artificial or replacement body part.

Quadrantectomy An operation that removes a quarter of the breast.

Radiologist A specialist who takes and reads X-rays.

Radiotherapist A specialist who gives radiotherapy.

Tumor A new lump, which can be benign or malignant.

Wide excision Cutting out a lump with a minimum of 1 centimeter of tissue around it.

USEFUL ADDRESSES

BREASTFEEDING

La Leche League of Canada
18C Industrial Drive
P.O. Box 29
Chesterville
ON K0C 1H0
Tel: (613) 448 1842
Fax: (613) 448 1845
Mother to mother breastfeeding help, information, and resource centre

BREAST CARE

Marvelle Koffler Breast Centre
Mount Sinai Hospital
600 University Avenue
Toronto
ON M5G 1X5
Tel: (416) 586 5065
Fax: (416) 586 8555
An integrated, comprehensive breast care centre

Henrietta Banting Breast Centre
Women's College Hospital
60 Grosvenor Street
Toronto
ON M5S 1B2
Tel: (416) 323 6400 ext. 4424
Fax: (416) 323 7314
Multidisciplinary care for patients with breast problems

Regional Women's Health Clinics
Contact your local Health Centre or doctor for the Regional Women's Health Clinic nearest you

Regional Women's Health Centre, Toronto
790 Bay Street, 8th Floor
Toronto
ON M5G 1N9
Tel: (416) 586 0211
      (416) 351 3716 (Library)
Resource and counselling centre for women's concerns

Breast Screening Program
Friendly, easily accessible centres for women aged 50 or over in which to receive mammograms, physical examination of the breast, and instruction about breast self-examination from trained health care professionals. Offered by British Columbia,
Alberta, Saskatechewan, Ontario, Nova Scotia, and the Yukon, and currently being set up in other provinces. The following phone numbers will connect you to the nearest Breast Screening Program:

British Columbia
1-800 663 9203

Alberta
1-800 667 0604

Saskatchewan
1-800 667 0017

Ontario
1-800 668 9304

Nova Scotia
1-902 428 5960

Yukon
(403) 668 6252

CANCER

Canadian Cancer Society
10 Alcorn Avenue, Suite 200
Toronto
ON M4V 3B1
Tel: (416) 961 7223
Fax: (416) 961 4189
Provides a variety of support programs and educational resources for cancer patients and their families

Breast Cancer Society of Canada
401 St Clair Street
Point Edward
ON N7V 1P2
Tel: (519) 336 0746
Fax: (519) 336 6846
National non-profit charitable organization dedicated to improving detection, prevention, and treatment of breast cancer

Canadian Breast Cancer Network
P.O. Box 45115
2482 Yonge Street
Toronto
ON M4P 2H0
Tel: (416) 244 1443
Fax: (416) 244 2363
E-Mail: stefhall@interlog.com
National network of groups and individuals to support people living with breast cancer

BREAST PROSTHESES

Ontario Ministry of Health
Prosthetics Consultant
Assistive Devices Program
5700 Yonge Street, 7th Floor
North York
ON M2M 4K5
Tel: (416) 327 8804
      1-800 268 6021
Provides assistance and funding

Breast Implant Line of Canada
56 Touraine Avenue
North York
ON M3H 1R2
Tel: (416) 636 6618
Fax: (416) 636 3570

GENERAL

A Friend Indeed Publications Inc.
Box 515
Place du Parc Station
Montreal
QC H2W 2P1
Tel: (514) 843 5730
Provides a newsletter for women in the prime of life

The Canadian Academy of Homeopathy
P.O. Box 357
Grimsby
ON L3M 4H8
Will help you find a certified homeopath

The Canadian Naturopathic Association
P.O. Box 4520
Station C
Calgary
AB T2T 5N3
Tel: (403) 244 4487
Fax: (403) 244 2340

The Sex Information and Education Council of Canada (SIECCAN)
850 Coxwell Avenue
East York
ON M4C 5R1
Tel: (416) 466 5304

INDEX

ACKNOWLEDGMENTS

MEDICAL CONSULTANT
Professor R.E. Mansel MS FRCS

ADVICE AND ASSISTANCE
Breast Cancer Care; Dr. Helena Earl, University Hospital Birmingham; Mr. J.D. Frame FRCS, FRCS (Plast); Mr. Jerry Gilmore MS, FRCS, FRCS (Ed.); Dr. Eleanor Moskovic MRCP, FRCR, The Royal Marsden NHS Trust; National Childbirth Trust; National Screening Co-ordination Office; Angela O'Grady, King's College Hospital; Patricia Paniale, Royal Free Hampstead NHS Trust; Professor R.D. Rubens MD, BSc, FRCP, Guy's Hospital; Professor John Sloane, University of Liverpool; Twins and Multiple Births Association

TYPESETTING
Debbie Lelliott, Axis Design

FILM OUTPUT
Disk To Print (UK) Ltd

CLOTHING AND EQUIPMENT
Rigby and Peller, London (bras); The Bullen Health Care Group, Manchester (prostheses); Nicola Jane, Chichester (prostheses)

ADDITIONAL EDITORIAL ASSISTANCE
Jennifer Rylaarsdam

ADDITIONAL DESIGN ASSISTANCE
Helen George

PROOFREADER
Lesley Ward

INDEX
Barbara Hird

ANATOMICAL REFERENCES
Sandie Hill

ILLUSTRATIONS AND CHARTS
Tony Graham: pp.37, 38, 39, 40, 41, 79, 132, 148, 155, 157, 160, 162, 180, 191
Paul Williams: pp.42, 61, 62, 74, 94, 109, 110, 112, 116, 117, 121, 122, 123, 124, 125, 127, 128, 129, 135, 141, 142, 146, 151, 159, 161, 178

PICTURE RESEARCH
Sandra Schneider

PICTURE CREDITS
Archaeological Museum, Aleppo p.72; Breast Screening Unit, King's College Hospital/Science Photo Library (SPL) pp.7, 115, 127 (top right), 130, 131, 137; Christie's, London/Bridgeman Art Library, London p.20 (bottom left); Collections/Anthea Sieveking p.100; Werner Forman Archive p.15; Dr. Rosalind Given-Wilson, Consultant Radiologist, St. George's Hospital NHS Trust p.48 (center left); Sarah Errington/The Hutchison Library p.88; E.T. Archive/National Museum, Athens p.70; Mary Evans Picture Library pp.8, 20 (top right and bottom right), 21 (top and bottom right); Mr. J. D. Frame pp.109, 190; Stephen Gerard/SPL pp.7, 11, 65 (top); Images Colour Library pp.5, 19; King's College School of Medicine, Department of Surgery/SPL p.45 (center); King's College School of Medicine/SPL pp.48 (center right and right), 158; The Kobal Collection p.28; Kunsthistorisches Museum, Vienna/Bridgeman Art Library, London p.17; Louvre, Paris/Giraudon/Bridgeman Art Library, London p.16; Niall McInerney p.71 (top); Dr. P. Marazzi/SPL pp.63, 134 (bottom); M. Marshall, Custom Medical Stock Photo/SPL p.112 (top right); Eleanor Moskovic, The Royal Marsden NHS Trust pp.48 (left), 139, 157, 161 (bottom), 175, 181; National Gallery, London/ Bridgeman Art Library, London p.20 (top left); National Medical Slide Bank pp.45 (top), 110 (bottom left and right), 112 (bottom left and right), 134 (top), 136; Joseph Nettis/SPL p.184; Dr. Heather Nunnerley, Director of Radiology, King's College Hospital, London p.133; Popperfoto p.34; Prado, Madrid/Bridgeman Art Library, London pp.6, 13, 14; Chris Priest/SPL pp.65 (bottom left), 127 (bottom left and bottom right); Range/Bettmann/UPT p.23; Mr. N. P. M. Sacks, Consultant Surgeon and Head of Breast Unit, St. George's Hospital NHS Trust p.108; Professor John Sloane, University of Liverpool p.156; Tony Stone Images p.65 (bottom right); Tate Gallery, London p.71 (bottom); Victoria and Albert Museum, London/Bridgeman Art Library, London p.21 (bottom left); ZEFA pp.30, 46

MODELS
Kareen Aliane; Annalisa Bacchi; Helena Bridge and Susanna; Claire Farman, James Catto, and India Rose; Wendy Nehorai; Ana Rizzo

MAKEUP
Bettina Graham

AUTHOR PHOTOGRAPH
(back jacket flap)
Slater King